THE MISWIRED CHILD

HOW MODERN CHILDHOOD HARMS THE BRAIN

DR. KIMBERLY IDOKO

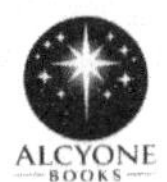

ALCYONE
BOOKS

CONTENTS

Alcyone Books

This book is for informational and educational purposes only. It is not intended as a substitute for professional legal advice, medical advice, diagnosis, or treatment. Always seek the advice of qualified professionals regarding your specific condition or concern.

Hardcover ISBN: 979-8-9943406-0-8

Paperback ISBN: 979-8-9943406-1-5

E-book ISBN: 979-8-9943406-2-2

Audio ISBN: 979-8-9943406-3-9

1st Edition, April 2026

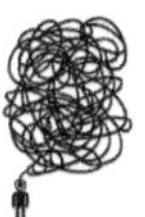

DEDICATION

To every parent who can't afford to look away.

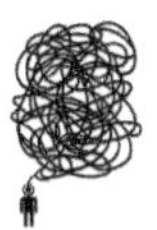

PREFACE

There's a moment every parent remembers. Maybe you're watching your child repeat a flicker, a gesture, or a stillness, and your stomach drops. Something clenches inside before you can name what you're feeling, because some part of you already knows.

You see it first.

Later, you're alone in the kitchen, scrolling through symptoms you wish you hadn't found, searching for comfort you wish you didn't need. The moment has lodged itself in the body. It draws a line through time, and everything arranges itself as before or after: before the white coat, before the care plan. For many parents, it's also the last moment they fully trust their own eyes.

What follows looks like help. A rush of referrals, a cascade of therapies, instructions about what to accept and what to track and what to work on. Sometimes it even sounds like hope. But the part no one names is the biology that shifted long before any diagnosis arrived. Biology always shifts first.

Here's the truth to hold from the start: the way through begins by seeing what's real, not by digging through jargon or waiting for science to hand you permission. Before symptoms draw attention, something quieter is already changing inside the brain. Networks that hold speech, focus, memory, and mood begin to lose resilience. A single gene can light the fuse, but a harsh environment is what keeps it burning. This is where collapse takes root, long before anyone is looking.

This book is about what precedes that collapse. I call it miswiring: the unraveling before the screaming starts, before the light dims, before the paperwork begins. It's about what builds a brain and what sabotages it, and about what happens when surface symptoms are mistaken for roots.

I write about this as a mother, and also as a board-certified neurologist and children's rights attorney who has seen, time and again, what happens when evidence bends and policy fails the most vulnerable.

I was four years old when I was shot. A bullet fired by accident shattered my sense of safety, and it lit a fire in me to understand the body: how it breaks and how it heals. I skipped grades, devoured math and science, and chased frameworks that could hold chaos. That hunger carried me to Yale, where I fell in love with neurobiology, then to the University of Pennsylvania to master medicine, then to Stanford Law to study how industry, regulation, and policy intertwine and how evidence can bend to serve profit over people.

Along the way came heaps of praise, but threaded through it was a hollow truth: I still didn't quite know what real health required. When my son was born, everything followed the textbooks, and that orderly arrival brought with it a false assurance that I had what I needed.

Then came my daughter. By two, she was diagnosed with autism. By three, Rett syndrome. Suddenly every forkful of food, every shift in sleep, and every flicker of skill or loss carried enormous weight. Just like that, I entered a world I had no training for.

On one side, clinicians offered data but no hope. On the other, influencers promised miracles through celery juice and detox protocols. In between stood me: a neurologist grounded in evidence, a parent praying for possibility, a woman staring into the space between what's known and what's possible. That desperation broke me open.

I returned to the literature, moving through neurology, nutrition, immunology, and physiology, studying the roots of healing. The cellular kind that unfolds when conditions are right, rather than the curated kind that sells supplements. In the fog, I found discernment. In the rubble, I found direction. And I stopped chasing magic.

But this book reaches beyond one child's diagnosis and one mother's discernment. It's about the constant collision of fragile wiring with careless systems, and about how parents are repeatedly asked to trust structures that profit from delay. Waiting is where neurons die. Load accumulates long before the next well-child visit, and injury deepens long before the next referral. Once you see both the biology and the betrayal, the world looks different and stays that way.

If you've ever been told to "wait and see," you know the particular ache of that delay. If you've ever been told your child's struggles were "just anxiety" or "strong will," you know the chasm between what you witnessed and what got dismissed. If you've ever left a healthcare visit carrying more questions than you arrived with, this book is already yours.

The story you were given was incomplete, and your instincts were telling you something real. We've been trained to monitor the wrong things, to count words and chase milestones, to scan for disorder rather than distress, to defer to the plan and trust the experts and accept the reassurance. Meanwhile, five powerful systems muddy the terrain we're forced to cross. Big Food floods children's bodies with synthetic fuel. Big Pharma sells control instead of repair. Big Medicine chases symptoms and misses the roots beneath them. Big Government fails to guard the inputs that matter most. Big Media warps truth for clicks. Together these systems manufacture and amplify brain damage while convincing parents to look away.

This book is an autopsy of a society that keeps mistaking collapse for coincidence. It exists to name the betrayal and to trace how each system plays its part in miswiring our children.

I won't hand you a framework or a protocol. I'll hand you biology, and I'll walk you back to where your own answers begin.

But first, return to that moment. The one when your child did something that stopped time, something you couldn't explain and couldn't forget. That was the beginning, long before someone said "let's just monitor" and long before any diagnosis. That flicker was your child's body begging for steadiness. Even when no one else saw it, you did.

You still do. Hold on to that.

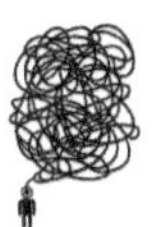

INTRODUCTION

The waiting room hums with the particular quiet of people bracing themselves. Plastic chairs line the walls, the air carries the scent of disinfectant and coffee gone cold, and somewhere across the room a clock marks time. Every parent in that room knows the feeling: the internal alarm when something in a child changes and won't change back.

It always starts small. A baby who once slept deeply now startles awake, eyes wide, as if her own brain won't let her rest. A toddler who babbled freely now grasps at sounds that stall halfway. A preschooler who once moved through the day with ease now erupts over nothing and then collapses in your arms.

It's tempting to explain it away: teething, temperament, a phase. You repeat what you've been told. But something in your chest isn't buying it. Your body tenses in waiting rooms. Your gut tightens when reassurance comes too fast. Your mind searches for proof to quiet what your instincts already know, so you start looking: late at night on your phone, in whispers with other parents, everywhere. What comes back is noise. One voice says it's normal. Another says act now. Another blames your parenting. None of it fits your child.

The system speaks in ranges and percentiles. Your child

speaks in patterns: what changes first, what changes next, and what doesn't return. Those two languages rarely line up, and that mismatch is the opening crack.

Long before anyone reaches for a checklist, parents feel the shift. Days gain weight. Nights stretch thin. A child who once moved easily through the world now strains against it, energy thinning, reserves running close to empty. What appears minor is often the first sign of biology working harder than it should.

It starts with load. A young brain takes in more than it can repair, and that imbalance, small at first, repeats. The body adjusts, then over-adjusts. Sleep stops restoring. A child's spark flickers from pressure building where no one is looking.

Think of Mateo, age three. He used to sing in the bath and name every dog on the block. Over a few months, the songs fade, words slip, and naps crumble. He spins the wheels of a toy car and looks through you, a subtle dimming that only his mother sees. She's told to wait; her body says don't.

Picture their house at two in the morning. The hallway light is soft. The fridge hums. She stands in his doorway, watching him rock, and she knows something has shifted. That shift is real.

Miswiring is invisible until it isn't. A child can pass screenings and still be unraveling. They can charm a teacher while their brain strains to hold the day together. They can look entirely typical while something deeper is changing in ways no chart reflects. Our culture names what's obvious and rarely asks what's happening beneath it.

Parents often sense these early signals. They notice when the day starts to fray. They recognize patterns others dismiss. Sometimes they're told they're anxious or dramatic, and that dismissal becomes its own injury. When nothing gets named, parents begin doubting the one thing that's been accurate from the start: their own knowing.

But miswiring has a shape. It has drivers. It has early signs. And it responds to the same truths biology has always responded to: steadier fuel, deeper rest, safer rhythm, fewer hits to fragile circuits.

This book offers you a clearer lens. In the pages ahead, you'll see how load accumulates quietly, how small losses in rhythm and repair set the stage long before anything looks dramatic. You'll see why children buckle when thresholds are crossed and why progress can rise and fall without warning. You'll see early signals move across sleep, focus, and stamina in ways systems don't track. You'll see why labels never felt complete, why waiting felt dangerous, and why your instincts kept circling the same small details.

By the end, you'll see your child differently. The meltdown after the classroom treat won't be a mystery. The blank stare at four in the afternoon will make sense. The night waking won't feel like bad luck. You'll recognize the pattern, and more importantly, you'll know where to intervene.

You'll see yourself differently too. Your unease was data, not weakness. Your intuition was the earliest, most accurate signal in the room.

The promise here is clarity, not a quick fix. Clarity breaks the fog and steadies your next step, and it protects your child from systems that weren't built to see them. Biology has rules. Once you understand them, the path forward comes into view.

PART 1
MISWIRING
WHERE COLLAPSE BEGINS

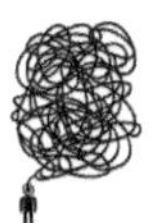

CHAPTER 1

THE BLIND SPOT

MISWIRING hides well because five systems depend on that blindness. Big Food drains children's biology from the inside out. Big Pharma manages the fallout. Big Medicine breaks the story into disconnected parts. Big Government funds the fragments and calls it a system. Big Media tells families they're worrying too much. Each one benefits when fragile wiring gets mistaken for choice, and together they've built a world that rewards that mistake.

The people inside these systems are mostly not villains. They're physicians who trained inside institutions that reward speed over pattern, researchers who study what funders prioritize, regulators who interpret rules shaped by the industries they oversee, and journalists chasing the story that travels fastest. Individual integrity exists everywhere in this landscape, and it matters. The problem is structural: incentives that reliably produce the same outcomes whether or not anyone intends them. That's what makes the blind spot so durable. It runs on a system optimized for the wrong things, and a system like that reproduces itself without anyone having to choose it.

Our tools don't catch miswiring because they weren't built to.

They pick up problems late, charts sorting children into tidy boxes and calling it insight, screenings skimming the surface and missing the pressure rising underneath, labels freezing a moving process and declaring the job done, explaining how to file rather than why a child is struggling in the first place. When institutions stop at symptoms, parents are left managing what's visible while the invisible keeps steering the day.

Before naming miswiring, it helps to name what it isn't, because the cultural story around it has been wrong for a long time. Miswiring isn't character. It isn't temperament, and it certainly isn't a parenting failure. It's demand outrunning supply: a young brain carrying more than its cells can restore, a body asking for steadiness so repair can begin.

When a depleted child gets mistaken for a stubborn one, blame falls on them. When a fragile system gets mistaken for personality, the struggle looks permanent. When miswiring gets pinned on the home, guilt buries truth. Seen clearly, miswiring is none of those things. It's physiology.

Some children inherit thinner margins. Their wiring starts life already under tension. But genes only set the opening conditions. What happens next depends on the world that meets them: food, sleep, stress, light, noise. The same daily load another child absorbs can push this one past capacity. Miswiring isn't one event. It's accumulation, the process by which ordinary life turns into overload.

From the outside, a child can look completely typical, milestones met, teachers charmed, days held together by sheer effort. Meanwhile, inside the body, repair falls behind and strain builds layer by layer. Miswiring stays quiet until the system can't compensate anymore. Then signals appear: stamina thinning, sleep growing fragile, focus shattering, mood slipping, movement unable to settle. These are physiology asking for help, not quirks.

Parents notice these shifts because they're living beside the child every day. They see which moments wobble, which tasks drain, which days cost more than they should. These early changes sketch the full story long before any number does. But systems built to read data points can't register patterns. Delay gets disguised as reassurance, and language finishes the job. Systems speak in categories rather than causes, and categories keep things tidy for institutions while miswiring lives in exactly the details those categories erase. So symptoms get catalogued while the forces driving them go unnamed, and families are told to manage the label while the root stays untouched.

Families feel that blind spot directly. They adjust routines, try charts, firmer limits, softer voices. When nothing holds, self-doubt moves in, and that doubt becomes part of the injury. Once miswiring is named, though, blame quiets and curiosity begins. The question shifts from "Why is my child like this?" to "What's asking for steadiness that isn't getting it?" Under strain, the whole system moves into protection mode, and what looks like willfulness or withdrawal is often conservation. When stability returns, a child learns, regulates, and adapts.

Parents don't need another theory of childhood. They need a lens that restores cause and effect, and miswiring offers exactly that. It reveals what's been hiding in plain sight: a body rationing energy while institutions call the signals misbehavior, mood, or temperament. Systems that should detect strain have instead built normalcy around it, teaching parents to mute the very signs that point toward where help is needed. That confusion is structural. Our economy rewards reaction over prevention and silence over pattern.

Once you see miswiring, the fog lifts. You stop chasing labels and start decoding, stop bracing for crisis and start noticing in real time, stop asking whether you're overreacting and start asking where your child's system is losing ground.

Set aside the story that treats adaptation as design. Set aside the suggestion that this is simply who your child is. Set aside any timeline that tells you to wait while a harsh world teaches the wrong lessons to a nervous system already stretched thin.

Replace all of it with a clearer truth: this is capacity under pressure, measurable across time and describable without blame.

Once miswiring comes into view, everything shifts. You see the difference between won't and can't. Right now, your child can't. And delay leaves marks.

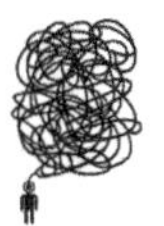

CHAPTER 2

CELLULAR DISRUPTION

COLLAPSE BEGINS QUIETLY, long before the signs make sense.

Long before sleep breaks down or focus slips, something inside each cell starts falling out of rhythm. The shift is tiny and silent, but the body feels it.

Think of a cell as a small city. It feeds itself, clears waste, repairs damage, and keeps its lights on moment by moment. When supplies are steady and defenses hold, the city hums along. When those supply lines thin, everything slows. Machinery runs longer than it should. Waste lingers and corners dim.

Collapse starts there, in the timing of repair rather than in how a child looks.

At first, the slowdown hides well. A child still laughs, runs, and learns. The spark stays, just softer. The body covers the gaps today by borrowing from tomorrow. Parents may notice the bedtime that drags out, the fragile morning, the sudden mood drop with no clear trigger. These are signals from tiny cities running low.

Modern life feeds that strain. Food built for shelf life rather than biology. Air carrying chemicals too small to see. Noise that never settles. Screens that shine long after night should begin. None of these alone breaks a system, but together they stall the very repairs a developing brain depends on. Disruption piles up slowly until there's no way to hide it. A whisper repeated becomes a warning.

Inside those cities, communication slows. Messages that once traveled cleanly now crawl. Energy dips and the system talks in static. The brain tries to make sense of that static, and the effort shows up as irritability, fatigue, fog, or restlessness. From the outside it looks emotional. From the inside it's electrical.

Children feel this loss of rhythm sharply because their cells are still building the structures they need for learning and growth. Every developmental leap depends on timing inside those cities. When timing slips or fuel runs low, learning feels harder, attention shorter, calm farther away. What a teacher calls distractibility is often a body stretching its last reserves.

You've seen the shape of it long before anyone names it. Days go sideways after certain meals or broken sleep. A crash follows an overstimulating afternoon. Weeks arrive when nothing holds and your child seems distant from themselves. Biology always speaks, just quietly at first.

Parents rarely get taught this translation. You're told to manage what's visible without understanding what's invisible, even though the invisible is where the story begins. Once you understand that every vacant stare or sudden burst of motion is the body reporting its own conditions, the question shifts from "What's wrong with my child?" to "What is my child's body trying to say?"

Disruption doesn't need catastrophe to take hold. It grows through small things: missed nutrients, short nights, stress that never fully clears. A child can endure those conditions for a while. Building well inside them is another matter. Over time, tiny deficits accumulate.

A developing brain protects itself first. When energy is tight, it dims higher functions so the basics can hold. Patience, focus, and social ease are expensive capacities, and they're the first to fade so the foundation can stay stable. It's allocation: the body guarding itself one circuit at a time.

Understanding this changes everything. You stop judging outward behavior and start listening underneath it. You stop asking for performance from a system that's signaling distress. You begin reading every meltdown or foggy moment as a flare from the smallest units of life, asking for steadiness.

Parents who learn this language become fluent in prevention. They stop chasing labels and start tracing causes. They watch patterns rather than isolated moments. They notice the body's ongoing conversation with its world: mornings versus afternoons, how mood shifts with meals, how sleep predicts the next day's stability.

Clarity doesn't fix everything, but it ends the confusion that makes everything harder.

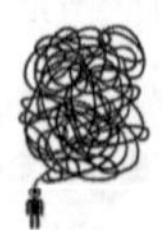

CHAPTER 3

THE BODY'S FIRST LANGUAGE

BEFORE WORDS, before diagnosis, a child's biology is already speaking. It speaks in hunger and calm, in motion and stillness, in color and tone. Every cell sends signals upward, electrical and chemical messages reporting one essential condition: whether the environment feels stable enough to grow.

When that conversation runs clean, development holds its rhythm. Sleep deepens, appetite arrives on time, curiosity comes online, and energy rises and falls in predictable arcs. The body moves through effort and recovery without friction. When the system strains, the language changes. Signals cross, meaning blurs, and static enters the line.

You see it in the child who can't settle, who keeps moving because stillness exposes fragility. In the one who fades early, the spark gone by noon. In the quiet child whose gaze slides past you, retreating from load rather than from disinterest. Each pattern is a dialect of the same truth: the body's no longer at ease.

Every symptom belongs to a vocabulary. Some children speak through skin, rashes flaring when immune signaling runs hot or barriers falter. Others speak through movement, through voices that rise, through sleep that won't arrive. Some speak through retreat, the silence of circuits protecting themselves. What looks like quirk or personality is structured communication from a system under strain.

We once read this language instinctively. Long before charts and checklists, caregivers watched posture, breath, skin temperature, appetite, the quality of a cry. That literacy kept children alive. Modern life didn't erase the language so much as change what gets rewarded. Quiet became success. Endurance became virtue, and a child could appear regulated while quietly paying a steep internal cost.

Silence can be camouflage, and the body keeps its own timing regardless of whether anyone's reading it. Symptoms appear with consistency long before they're named. Meltdowns crest at the same hour. Fatigue arrives before dinner every night. Focus dissolves after certain foods or certain rooms. These repetitions are physiology replaying the same conditions against the same limited reserve, and they carry pattern long before they carry a label.

When adults interpret these signals as attitude or temperament, the story distorts. A child gets labeled oppositional instead of overloaded, a crash gets called laziness instead of depletion, and a shutdown gets mistaken for calm. The labels describe appearance rather than mechanism, and the body keeps responding anyway.

Once symptoms are understood as language, mystery narrows. What once felt chaotic begins to organize, and the same signals line up in sequence. The child stops looking unpredictable and starts looking consistent, consistent in response to consistent inputs. That's the turning point, a shift in frame: the child's body is responding to conditions, not choosing chaos.

The question beneath every symptom, every withdrawal, every surge is the same one: what's feeding it?

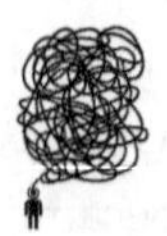

CHAPTER 4

ENERGY AND THE CHILD'S BRAIN

EVERY SIGNAL, every emotion, every bit of learning runs on energy. A child's brain is the hungriest organ in the body, burning fuel at a rate that would exhaust an adult. Growth is a sustained electrical storm, and every thought, movement, and adjustment draws current. When that current is steady, development feels almost effortless: words form, focus holds, sleep restores, and a child moves through effort and recovery without friction, curiosity coming online and receding again as it should. When the current falters, everything costs more. Circuits blink, mood shortens, and learning turns uphill as the brain starts asking for power it doesn't have.

Energy is the foundation most systems never name. Behavior gets corrected and performance gets rewarded, but the fuel that makes performance possible rarely gets examined. Yet every outward expression, attention, movement, emotion, is only the surface of an internal economy.

The body budgets energy across growth, repair, learning, and defense. When supply runs thin, it reallocates, and that reallocation follows biology rather than preference. The body first protects what keeps the organism alive and trims what looks optional. Patience fades first, then flexible attention, then social ease, and what remains is often motion without modulation or stillness without engagement. From the outside, these look like extremes. From the inside, they're conservation.

A child low on energy doesn't always resemble an exhausted adult. Many look restless, because the nervous system pushes movement to stay alert when stillness exposes the deficit. Output rises as the body leans on stress chemistry to hold itself upright, and the pacing, the climbing, the talking, the crashing are the nervous system attempting to compensate for a power shortage. Other children move in the opposite direction: speech thins, eyes lose depth, and the system pulls back to protect what remains as engagement becomes expensive and presence fades. Different expressions, same math. Demand has exceeded supply, and the brain is adjusting to survive it.

Modern childhood drains energy faster than many developing systems can restore it. Meals engineered for convenience rather than repair, nights shortened by artificial light and noise, days spent in environments that keep bodies in low-grade vigilance: none of these alone breaks a system, but together they erode reserve until the brain begins rationing as a long-term strategy.

Inside that rationing, higher functions grow fragile. The brain prioritizes maintenance over synthesis and can't integrate new information while it's working just to hold its baseline stable. Reasoning disappears mid-storm, attention collapses after overstimulation, and memory slips on depleted days. What gets labeled inconsistency is the nervous system fluctuating around a shrinking margin.

When the energy economy stays negative, biology changes priorities. Growth slows, repair defers, and stress chemistry stops being an emergency response and becomes a standing tool. Research in children and adults consistently shows that chronic energy deficits shift the nervous system toward patterns that favor vigilance and endurance over flexibility and learning. The brain adapts to what it perceives as an unstable environment, and those adaptations show up in behavior long before they show up on any chart. What once required rest now requires effort. What once recovered overnight now lingers. Capacity narrows without announcement.

Here's what's worth holding carefully: the brain's capacity for adaptation runs in both directions. The same plasticity that allows a stressed nervous system to reorganize around scarcity also allows it to reorganize toward recovery when conditions improve. Wiring that formed under pressure responds to steadier inputs, and that responsiveness is the foundation everything else in this book builds on. The pivot most adults miss is this: the system has been running a reasonable adaptation to unreasonable conditions, and reasonable adaptations can change when the conditions do.

Energy is constraint. It determines how much function is available, how much recovery is possible, and how close the system is to its threshold. In a developing brain, that margin matters more than output because it decides whether wiring builds forward or folds inward. Long before anything looks dramatic, the system is already making compromises, and those compromises accumulate without announcing themselves, surfacing only when the margin is gone.

Energy first. Function second. This is how brains are built.

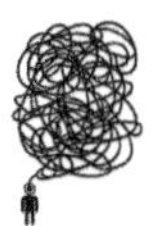

CHAPTER 5

THE TIPPING POINT

FOR A WHILE, the body absorbs disruption and keeps going. It adjusts, compensates, and hides strain behind function. Then one day the math stops working. Repair costs more than it restores, and the body crosses a line it can't uncross on its own.

Collapse gathers like pressure behind a dam. Each stress, each toxin, each broken night adds a drop. The wall holds, hairline cracks forming quietly, and the child keeps smiling, keeps learning, keeps almost keeping up. Then something small, a fever, an antibiotic, a hard week at school, lands on weight already there, and the structure gives way.

Parents can often name the moment. The morning their child's voice changed. The week their eyes lost light. The night sleep broke and never quite found its rhythm again. Medicine calls it regression. The truth is simpler and harder to sit with: the body reached its threshold. The energy economy collapsed. What once looked like resilience was exhaustion wearing a familiar face.

At that point, biology changes priorities. Cells stop investing in growth and shift toward protection. Circuits that once reached forward begin to pull back. Signaling slows. Repair slips behind schedule. The system that once buffered strain discreetly now broadcasts it through irritability, anxiety, fog, and withdrawal. Each is a flare. The message is blunt: I can't buffer this anymore.

This is where misunderstanding compounds harm. The flares get labeled instead of interpreted. Teachers call them acting out. Clinicians adjust medications. Everyone explains the surface and no one names the threshold. The body has been saying it's at capacity, and the room keeps replying: try harder.

Before collapse becomes obvious, the body negotiates fiercely. It reallocates nutrients, slows growth, and leans on stress hormones to hold performance together. Decline hides behind effort. Parents see storms that come too easily and recovery that takes too long. Instinct says the wall is cracking, and that instinct is rarely acknowledged until the wall gives way.

Once it does, the pattern shifts fast. The child who managed transitions now panics at small changes. The one who loved reading can't find words. Sleep fragments. Appetite fades. The body stops cycling and starts looping, trying to stay afloat on what energy remains.

This is the tipping point, the moment parents feel the ground move beneath them. Their child's biology has reorganized around depletion, and adaptation has turned into injury.

Mechanisms that once protected begin to harm. Alarms stay on even when danger has passed. Inflammation rises. Survival takes the lead. Strategies that once worked stop working, and the familiar world, where rest fixed fatigue and patience calmed storms, no longer applies.

This moment is the body drawing a boundary. Once seen, that boundary becomes a map.

The tipping point teaches two things: symptoms aren't random, and they stack. Sleep debt, nutrient loss, illness, chemical exposure: rarely a single cause, almost always layered. Each weight matters. Each one can be lowered.

When the structure fails, the path becomes visible. Trace it back.

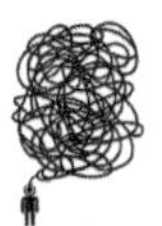

CHAPTER 6

WHEN THE BRAIN LOSES RHYTHM

AFTER THE TIPPING POINT, the brain's sense of order drifts. What once moved in sequence, waking, eating, learning, resting, loses its timing. Days stretch and nights fragment. The child keeps going, but their internal tempo no longer matches the world around them.

A healthy brain runs on rhythm. Hormones rise and fall on schedule. Body temperature shifts. Attention peaks and recedes. These cycles are instructions rather than habits or preferences. Rhythm tells the brain when to build, when to recover, when to be alert, and when to stand down. When timing holds, learning sticks, emotions stay proportionate, and the system knows where it is in the day.

Modern life disrupts that timing systematically. Activity stays high when the body expects release. Sleep starts later and ends earlier. Once cues blur, the brain starts guessing.

You see it in the child wide awake late at night and foggy by morning. In appetite that disappears or spikes at odd hours. In energy that surges just as the day should wind down. These are signs the internal clock has lost its reference point.

Inside the brain, timing is communication. Thousands of biological clocks coordinate everything from digestion to memory consolidation, and they rely on consistent cues, light, darkness, routine, to stay aligned. When those cues scatter, synchronization breaks. One system prepares for rest while another pushes for alertness, and what results is friction. Attention slips, mood swings, thought fragments, because the brain no longer knows when to regulate.

Rhythm is also how the body decides whether the world is safe. Predictable cycles signal stability. When effort reliably leads to rest, when hunger reliably meets nourishment, when night reliably brings sleep, the nervous system can stand down. When those sequences fall apart, it stays braced instead.

Without rhythm, signals overlap and the body's systems compete. Energy scatters instead of cycling. The child becomes wired and tired at the same time, too alert to rest, too depleted to engage.

This is a rhythm problem, not a mood problem or a discipline issue. When rhythm breaks, biology breaks with it. Growth stalls. The brain loses its place in the day, then its place in the body.

Rhythm is foundational. Adaptation has a cost.

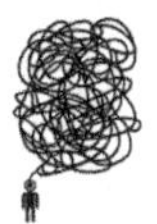

CHAPTER 7

THE HIDDEN COST OF SURVIVAL MODE

WHEN QUIET STOPS FEELING SAFE, the body starts scanning. Vigilance becomes the default state. The brain holds its guard up so long that rest begins to feel wrong and calm registers as threat. Survival mode is steady exhaustion, the body sleeping with its eyes open. Muscles stay half-tensed, ready for a signal that never resolves. Stress hormones meant for emergencies begin shaping ordinary days. The child who once recovered between stressors now lives inside the stress itself.

This state doesn't require catastrophe. Duration is enough. When timing stays broken, the body adapts to instability as if it's the environment. Motion starts to feel safer than stillness. Noise feels normal. Quiet feels suspicious.

Survival mode settles in through persistence, and once there, the brain reallocates resources. Energy that should support learning, curiosity, and connection diverts toward threat detection. Focus narrows and exploration shuts down. Even empathy fades, because it depends on feeling safe enough to register another person. The child who once played freely now startles easily. The one who laughed without effort now seeks control over small things. Their biology is doing exactly what survival requires.

Prolonged alert reshapes the brain. Tension becomes the baseline. Circuits for calm and exploration weaken from disuse while circuits for vigilance strengthen through repetition. That's why some children can't stop arguing, worrying, or moving: the nervous system has learned that staying activated is how it survives. What looks like resistance is strategy, the system preserving the only state that's kept it upright.

From the outside, behavior gets judged without context and effort gets demanded where capacity is missing. Inside the body, the experience is relentless. Heart rate stays elevated even at rest. Breathing stays shallow. Sensations blur together. Excitement and fear share the same chemistry. Regulation is unavailable because the system is locked in defense. Parents often feel this shift in the way joy takes effort, in the stiffness of a hug, in the way calm never quite lands. They try structure, rewards, and consequences. None of it lasts, because none of it tells the body it's safe.

Bodies can't learn while they're bracing. Survival mode is expensive. Stress chemistry keeps firing. Circulation favors muscle over digestion, alertness over repair. Energy gets burned maintaining defense instead of restoring tissue. A child may look functional while the body runs a deficit that deepens with time.

When energy is rationed for defense, the future narrows. Skills don't consolidate. Learning doesn't generalize. Growth comes in uneven bursts, brief gains followed by long plateaus or sudden losses. The body keeps choosing what's urgent over what's important, because urgency feels like life or death.

As this state persists, the nervous system loses flexibility. It can still escalate, but coming back down becomes a struggle. Small stressors trigger outsized responses because the margin for error is gone. Recovery takes longer and each demand leaves a deeper mark. That's why survival mode often masquerades as inconsistency. A child can hold it together in one setting and unravel in another. They can manage mornings and collapse by afternoon. They can perform briefly, then crash hard. What looks unpredictable is depletion revealing itself in waves.

Over time, defense stops being a response and becomes maintenance. Stress chemistry no longer spikes and resolves: it idles. Sleep loses depth and repair windows shrink. The system adapts to carrying load instead of clearing it. The cost is metabolic. Immune activity stays elevated. Digestion runs inefficiently. Energy production shifts toward short-term output instead of clean recovery. The body becomes very good at getting through the day and very bad at restoring itself afterward.

This is where confusion deepens. Adults see effort and assume capacity. They see survival and mistake it for resilience. Resilience replenishes. Survival consumes. One builds margin; the other erodes it. A nervous system living here can't afford curiosity. Anything unstructured threatens the guardrails that defense depends on. Control, sameness, and motion become stabilizers for a system running without reserve.

This is the trap of survival mode: it works just well enough to delay recognition. The child limps along and everyone waits, until the cost surfaces somewhere it can no longer be hidden.

Every child in survival mode is running the same program: stay alert, stay alive. The hidden cost is a life lived at half-presence. Energy meant for learning and joy gets burned on defense instead. When defense runs too long, someone pays. The bill always comes due.

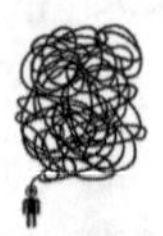

CHAPTER 8

THE UNSEEN INFLAMMATION

WHEN DEFENSE RUNS TOO LONG, chemistry changes.

The signals meant to protect the body don't shut off when danger passes. They linger. That lingering heat is inflammation, the quiet fire beneath modern childhood. It settles in, persistent and unresolved.

Inflammation is what happens when threat outlasts recovery. Each stress leaves a biochemical trace, a signal waiting for the next activation. When repair keeps pace, the body cools. When stress repeats faster than repair, cooling never completes. The fire stays lit, redirecting energy away from growth and toward containment. The body shifts from building to managing.

This state is often felt before it's measured. A child wakes heavy after a full night's sleep. Focus dissolves after meals. Tears arrive faster when sound rises. These are far more than personality traits or emotional quirks. They're thermal signals.

Inflammation lives in tissue long before it appears on paper.

Once established, inflammation tends to spread. It often begins in the gut, skin, or joints, where the signals are clearest and the triggers most direct. Research in both children and adults shows that sustained peripheral inflammation can affect brain function, slowing signaling, degrading timing, and contributing to the kind of mood and cognitive shifts that look behavioral from the outside. The precise mechanisms, and the degree to which they drive outcomes in children specifically, are still being mapped. What's already clear is the direction: when the body's inflammatory burden stays elevated, the brain operates in a noisier environment. A child forgets instructions halfway through, startles more easily, and loses access to ease. What gets mislabeled as bad behavior is often disrupted signaling working its way through an overloaded system.

What makes this state dangerous is its persistence. Inflammation doesn't need to be extreme to be disruptive. Low-grade heat, held long enough, degrades function. Repair keeps getting deferred. Recovery windows shrink. The body reorganizes around inflammation, prioritizing containment over capacity.

That adaptation has consequences. Learning grows fragile because consolidation depends on quiet chemistry. Growth slows because construction requires surplus energy. Exploration narrows because inflammation favors predictability over novelty. Biology begins choosing stability over expansion, not by preference but by necessity.

This is why survival mode and inflammation travel together. Defense chemistry stays active and immune signaling remains elevated. Energy meant for rebuilding never fully releases. The body becomes efficient at enduring demand and progressively worse at restoring itself afterward.

Inflammation also distorts perception. Hunger misfires. Fatigue arrives early. Sensory input overwhelms faster. Mood swings feel unprovoked because the margin for regulation has thinned. The body is reacting from a narrowed bandwidth.

Silence can be part of this picture too. A child who goes flat or withdraws may be conserving what little energy remains, their body occupied with managing internal heat. Expression becomes expensive. Calm, in this context, is load management.

This is where inflammation rewrites outcomes. A child may still function, but without reserve. Energy diverts from repair to containment, from integration to damage control. What's lost first is margin, and without it, development begins adapting downward to survive.

Inflammation follows pressure and it follows repetition. It's not random, and once established, it follows its own rules.

When the fire stays lit, capacity contracts. A body can survive in this state for a long time. It just can't develop there.

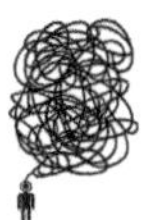

CHAPTER 9

THE SILENT CHILD

WHEN THE SMOKE CLEARS, the next phase is silence. The hollow kind that carries weight. The body is still there: warm skin, familiar eyes, a heartbeat that keeps time. But something inside the gaze has pulled back, as if presence itself has become too expensive.

It's recognized in contrast, not in comparison. What the child can no longer sustain becomes visible first. The laugh thins. The face stops rising to meet yours. The child who once reached without thinking now hovers at the edge of the room, close enough to touch, far enough to miss. It arrives as a series of small withdrawals rather than a single event, until stillness feels heavier than noise.

Distance is a metabolic decision.

A developing brain is a high-demand organ. Language, play, social attention, flexible movement, curiosity: these are energy-intensive functions. When the budget tightens, the brain triages. It protects the core and cuts the costliest operations first.

From the outside, it looks like loss. From the inside, it's conservation.

The shift is often misread because it isn't always loud. It can look tidy. Composed. A child who stops fighting a loud room may get praised for calming down. A child who stops reaching may get called easy. But this calm has a particular texture. In this state, the brain is minimizing output.

Eye contact slips because social processing is expensive. Speech thins because sequencing and retrieval draw heavily on strained reserves. Movement can turn repetitive because variation requires prediction, adjustment, and timing. The child isn't refusing connection. The brain is narrowing the channel to what it can afford.

The prevailing language frames this as a step backward. The physiology doesn't. What's happening is a reduction under pressure, not a return to an earlier state. Capacity falls and the nervous system reorganizes around survival arithmetic. When energy drops, the brain favors circuits that keep the organism intact and deprioritizes the circuits that make the child feel fully here, because those higher functions cost more.

Some children look as if they're underwater. Sound arrives late. Faces distort. Effort doubles. What once happened automatically now requires active, costly assembly. That's why words stop midstream. That's why laughter doesn't rise. That's why the body can move while the person feels distant. The brain is protecting fragile circuitry by lowering throughput.

The child who was overlays the child who remains while the world reaches for categories: delay, disorder, spectrum. These labels describe shape rather than load. They capture appearance while bypassing mechanism, a child withdrawing under strain.

Disappearance is an emergency posture. When the brain can't maintain stability, it reduces exposure and lowers demand. It dims the light to keep the bulb from shattering. The result can look like detachment, but it's protective. The nervous system is buying time.

Sometimes, without warning, fragments of connection return. A look. A sound. A reach. These moments feel miraculous because they arrive without notice or predictability, but they're physiology. They're the nervous system testing conditions, sampling whether it can spend without being punished for it. Every cell is listening for one message: that the world is stable enough to open again.

Those fragments don't mean the danger has passed. They mean capacity briefly rose or demand briefly fell.

What follows is a waiting period enforced by biology. In a developing brain, return isn't forced. It's permitted. Until capacity exceeds demand, higher circuits remain offline.

Silence isn't proof of healing. It's data.

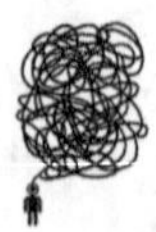

CHAPTER 10

WHEN THE WORLD DOESN'T BELIEVE YOU

THE MOMENT YOU NAME IT, resistance arrives.

Truth lands on the table and the room stills. Eyes drift to screens. Voices soften into professional phrases. "It's probably just a phase." "She just needs a little more structure."

You know otherwise.

Disbelief doesn't always shout. Sometimes it smiles, right before it hides behind developmental charts and normal ranges, thanks you for your concern, promises follow-up, and sends you home with paperwork that explains nothing. You leave carrying your child and something else the system added: doubt.

At first, you assume it's a misunderstanding. Maybe you didn't explain clearly enough. Maybe the timing was wrong. So you gather more notes, record more memories you can't shake, and try again. You speak calmly and carefully this time. The more specific you become, the more guarded the room grows. The more insistent you become, the smaller you feel in the chair across from authority.

"You're overthinking," they say. "Don't read so much online," they say. "Every child develops differently," they say. "Wait," they say.

Each phrase widens the distance between what you're seeing and what they're hearing.

Disbelief is structural. Waiting is wisdom. Delay is policy.

The clinicians delivering these phrases are rarely indifferent. Most of them chose this work because they wanted to help children. But they trained inside a system that rewards speed over pattern, that measures success in resolved complaints and clean charts, and that built the fifteen-minute visit as a feature rather than a flaw. Inside that architecture, a parent's nuanced, longitudinal knowledge of their specific child looks like noise. Dismissal isn't always a failure of character. Sometimes it's a failure of conditions, a physician with eighteen patients left in the afternoon and a screen demanding the next code, doing the best they can with a frame that was never wide enough to hold what you're carrying.

That distinction matters, because the parents who navigate this system most effectively are the ones who learn to work with the human inside the institution rather than against the institution itself. A clinician who feels interrogated closes. A clinician who feels like a partner opens. The same concern, delivered as an observation rather than an accusation, lands differently. Some still dismiss. But some pause, and that pause is where outcomes change.

Dismissing parents is easier than tracing early, subtle signals back to their roots. Rather than ask what disrupted a child's rhythm or what kept their brain in survival long enough to alter development, the system distorts the frame. It trains families to treat patterns as coincidence, to mistrust timing, to ignore repetition, and to doubt what happens after certain meals, in certain rooms, at certain hours.

Disbelief also turns parents into archivists. You build a case because the system requires one. Life reorganizes around proof and patterns become exhibits. The weight of proof becomes its own burden.

Bias sharpens the edge. Mothers are told that emotion clouds judgment, and when they cry, it confirms the suspicion. Fathers are urged to be rational, and when they push, they get labeled difficult. Both learn the same lesson: insistence is problematic, acceptance is virtue.

While adults debate thresholds and categories, the child's brain keeps wiring around strain. By the time the biology is too loud to ignore, the child has already been adapting for weeks, months, or years.

Inputs always land. Wiring follows.

None of this is accidental.

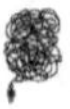

MISWIRING HAPPENS inside a body taking instructions all day long, and the first instructions arrive before symptoms do, before systems intervene, before anyone is looking. Food gets there first, most often, and with the least scrutiny. It teaches the nervous system what to expect, how to respond, and how much strain is normal. When those instructions destabilize energy, signaling, and repair, the brain adapts. That adaptation gets called coping until it gets called pathology.

Part Two begins where wiring meets its most constant influence.

PART 2
BIG FOOD

A SYSTEM, NOT A MEAL

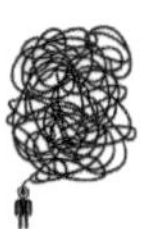

CHAPTER 11

FOOD IS INSTRUCTION

MORNING LIGHT SPILLS across the kitchen table. A spoon scrapes a bowl. A wrapper tears. Somewhere between one bite and the next, a child's body begins reading.

Each molecule carries a message. Some whisper calm and others shout confusion. Long before a child reads words, their cells are decoding chemistry. Food is instruction. When the brain reads clean code, in real protein, natural fat, and minerals that anchor enzymes, its choreography stays in sequence. Sleep restores, mood steadies, and circuits strengthen. When the code is corrupted by synthetic dyes, volatile sugars, and unstable oils, the translation breaks. The message becomes noise, and that noise lands as symptoms: sleep unraveling, focus scattering, tempers igniting then fading without reason. This is the body translating instructions.

The modern diet floods children with static: colorful cereals, squeezable yogurts, fortified snacks, juice boxes disguised as fruit. Marketing calls them balanced, but a developing brain hears interference. Neurons hungry for steady fuel can't keep time with volatility, so signals stutter and communication falters. The child doesn't describe it; they demonstrate it. A toddler wails through dinner, then collapses before bed. A kindergartener spins through recess, then crashes before pickup. A nine-year-old stares blankly at math that once made sense. Each of them is decoding chemistry that changes mid-sentence. This distortion is the product of a century that traded nourishment for convenience.

In the late 1940s, abundance met engineering. We had too much of certain raw ingredients, and industry learned to reshape them into something it called food. Mills turned grain into powder that stored. Refineries pulled sweetness into syrups. Presses drew oil from seeds that wouldn't spoil. Factories could bind, color, and flavor surplus into boxes that traveled farther than freshness ever could. Fortification became a promise stamped on the front while the kernel's life was stripped out inside. Labels promised balance while removing it. The message to parents was clear: if a box mentioned vitamins, its contents were welcome. By the 1960s, culture had learned to fear fat and forget nutrients. Sugar stepped in as the polite stand-in for pleasure. Breakfast shifted from eggs to aisles. Flavor grew louder as food grew thinner, and shelf life became the prize. By the time "kid food" appeared on shelves, culture was primed to believe children needed a separate diet, one engineered for influence rather than nourishment. Bright packaging, predictable sweetness, and textures that dissolved before they were chewed were among the earliest lessons in volatility. A developing brain learned to brace for the next surge.

In the late 1970s, the shift went national. Processed sweetness moved from commercials into cafeterias. The system framed it as preference. Biology experienced it as overload.

Inside every bite, instructions arrive. Some tell mitochondria to produce clean power and others ignite small fires of oxidation. The brain listens. Balanced signals stabilize neurotransmitters while chaotic ones unravel them. Parents see the difference: laughter to tears, focus to fog. Instability is often electrical. I remember an exam room where a mother spoke in patterns: after the classroom treat, he falls apart by pickup; after the brightly colored yogurt, he stops meeting my eyes by bath time. The chart was clean and the labs were normal, but the pattern held. Inputs predicted outcomes with metronomic accuracy.

Food sits on both axes. It can drive disruption or supply repair, corrode wiring or fund restoration. Genes set the margin, while environment decides whether the line gets crossed. For some children, that margin is narrow, with thresholds low and barriers thin. One snack may pass quietly through another child yet trigger days of volatility in this one. The difference is biology.

Every generation rewrites its definition of normal. We now call it typical for children to be restless, moody, sleepless, and distracted. We label fog as screen fatigue, meltdown as sensitivity, and collapse as personality. Yet these patterns rise with processed intake. The more the menu industrializes, the less the brain stabilizes. This is instruction scaled across a population.

The system still insists on neutrality. Boxes shout whole grain while stripped of minerals. Yogurts claim low sugar while sweetened with chemical cousins. Pediatric advice shrinks to growth charts and calories. What goes unspoken is this: the developing brain builds itself from what's eaten, molecule by molecule. Fortified sugar is still sugar. The child who unravels after snack time may be translating food into distress signals, and the system has no framework for that.

The cost of this silence shows up in classrooms and living rooms. What adults read as inattention, moodiness, or misbehavior is often something else entirely: biochemical confusion, circuits straining to find rhythm again. A child can memorize facts, maybe, but stability isn't something the brain manufactures from nothing. It has to be built from the right materials. Disorder repeated becomes disorder wired.

Food's betrayal is quiet because it's socially endorsed. The same ingredients that corrode neurons fund school fundraisers and pediatric conferences. The same flavors that destabilize attention fill lunch trays labeled balanced. Families trying to protect their children are told they're overreacting, and that's the oldest defense mechanism in any industry: mock the messenger until the message fades.

Most parents are simply choosing from what society has normalized, subsidized, advertised, celebrated, and placed directly into their children's hands through schools, pediatric offices, sports teams, and grocery aisles. Blame only makes sense when someone had a fair chance to see the truth, and most parents haven't, because the landscape is engineered to look safe.

Parents live the evidence anyway. They watch mornings that start bright dissolve after snacks. They watch evenings crash after sugar and weekends calm only when menus simplify. They start running experiments no study will ever fund: remove the dyes, delay the sugar, add protein first, then watch the body answer. The tragedy is that no one names this science. It gets called rigidity rather than research. Yet every observation fits the pattern of a nervous system reading its inputs. Every tantrum, fog, or sleepless night is data. A return of calm after steadier fuel is replication.

What's at stake is bigger than diet. It's agency. When a parent understands that food instructs, the power dynamic shifts. They stop being consumers of messaging and become interpreters of biology. They see that picky may be survival, a body rejecting volatility in the only way available to it. They see that kid food is a business model, not a need.

The developing body isn't sealed from the world. Its barriers are soft, its filters still forming. Every artificial input lands harder, stays longer, and writes deeper. That's why early exposure matters. That's why the same snack can change a day, and daily exposure can change a trajectory.

Science catches up slowly. But food is the script the brain learns from. Each meal teaches stability or chaos, coherence or confusion. You don't have to wait for consensus to notice. You only have to watch. The body tells the truth.

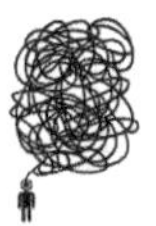

CHAPTER 12

KID FOOD IS CONDITIONING

THE PHRASE "KID FOOD" sounds harmless, almost tender. It conjures cartoon boxes, tiny forks, and plates that promise peace. It sells the illusion that childhood deserves its own cuisine: simpler, safer, sweeter. But kid food didn't evolve to nourish children. It evolved to capture them.

It began after the Second World War, when industry needed a market for cheap grain, sugar, and shelf-stable fats. Convenience was sold as modern freedom. As television took hold in the 1950s, advertising learned to bypass adults and target children directly. Cute jingles, mascots, toys in every box. Sugar became currency for compliance. Parents who served it were told they were efficient and modern. Behind the cartoon was a lab.

In the late 1970s, food technologists calibrated salt, sugar, and fat to hit the palate's sweet spot. Extruders puffed starch until it vanished on the tongue. Flavor houses built ripeness without fruit. Saturday mornings sold it. Schooldays sealed it. By the 1980s, a new rule had settled in: if it made children quiet, it must be valuable. Food became negotiation. Adults learned quickly which foods wouldn't cause a fight, and children adapted. Whole foods started arguments; processed foods ended them. Dinner battles were solved with beige nuggets and squeeze pouches. Breakfast tantrums softened with frosted cereals labeled "fortified," and nobody stopped to ask what they'd been fortified with, or at what cost. Industry had done its job. Parents were too reassured to question and too tired to resist.

In the 1990s, the costume changed but the chemistry didn't. "Lite," "low-fat," and "whole grain" claims multiplied while the ingredients stayed the same: refined starch padded with syrups, industrial fats chosen for shelf life, and colors brighter than anything a plant produces in nature. Parents were promised ease, and children were shaped by it.

Today, the design is even more precise. Every brightly packaged box runs on a sensory algorithm. Technologists test mouthfeel, crunch, and color saturation the way coders test software, with each iteration sharpening craving. Each bite trains expectation. Intensity becomes the reference point. A child hooked at two can become a lifelong customer by ten. This algorithm often eludes parents. They see twenty minutes of peace. A meal without tears. Relief. But what looks like calm is simply the chemistry settling for a moment.

Birthday parties, daycare menus, and school cafeterias all reinforce the same script: don't make food a fight, let kids be kids, moderation in all things. Meanwhile, the toddler rejects vegetables, the preschooler eats only beige, and the grade-schooler's moods spike and crash with sugar. Nobody questions why the menu for growing brains looks like a dessert aisle, because culture insists it's harmless tradition.

Parents who resist the script pay a social tax. A mother who removes dyes is told she's overreacting. A father who brings his own snacks is called obsessive. They're labeled rigid, controlling, or extreme, and that pressure to conform keeps the market stable. Each small surrender maintains the illusion of consensus. Parents try structure, then they try gentle. They're told they're too much, then told to relax. The system calls it choice: yogurts with cartoon faces, crackers fortified with calcium, nuggets shaped like dinosaurs. The same ingredients reappear under different labels, starch, oil, sugar, emulsifiers, and the palate narrows, the chemistry shifts, and the child miswires. In the quiet afterward, parents return to their kitchens lit by the glow of wrappers, wondering how something so basic slipped out of reach.

This is programming. Repeated exposure to engineered foods reshapes neural pathways, and the nervous system learns the wrong lessons. The brain that expects sweetness every few hours loses patience for subtlety. Dopamine spikes train anticipation. Attention shortens and self-regulation weakens. What looks like willpower failure is neurochemical adaptation, the early rehearsals for addiction. Each generation inherits a smaller definition of nourishment. The first was told to count calories. The next, to choose low-fat. Now parents are told to trust the box that says whole grain, even when it's mostly sugar.

The brain reads chemistry, not labels. It builds itself from whatever molecules are available. Children raised on engineered food learn two lessons: pleasure comes fast, and crashes follow. Their nervous systems adapt to volatility as baseline. What was once the brain's emergency mode, craving, surging, collapsing, becomes its daily pattern. The circuitry learns to chase stimulation. By adolescence, many children can't distinguish hunger from boredom, or exhaustion from overwhelm.

Parents who try to reintroduce real food are often met with resistance so strong it feels primal, because it is. Withdrawal looks like defiance. The body's learned dependency fights back.

This is the quiet violence of normalization. Industry calls it choice. Marketing calls it joy. Only later do parents see the cost.

Kid food is conditioning.

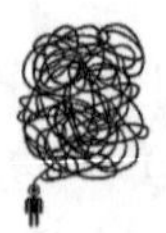

CHAPTER 13

CHILDHOOD IS POROUS

A TODDLER'S hand meets the world, then the mouth. The plastic toy, the carpet fiber, the crumb from breakfast. Each carries molecules small enough to slip through mucus and enter blood. Childhood is porous. Every touch is a transaction.

Early life moves fast. Neurons multiply, synapses connect and prune in waves, and development builds on itself. Yet the gates meant to protect that growth, the gut lining, immune network, and blood-brain barrier, are still under construction. They're scaffolds, not walls. The body is learning what to block and what to let through, and until that calibration finishes, everything in the environment auditions for permanence.

Think of these defenses as mortar that hasn't set. The gut learns to tell friend from foe. The immune system learns tolerance before it learns aggression. The brain's filter, the blood-brain barrier, learns to block noise from crossing into circuits. It's a beautiful choreography when timing holds, but modern life interrupts the rehearsal. Each exposure adds noise: dyes activating immune cells, emulsifiers associated with changes in gut lining integrity, sugars swinging metabolism, pollutants irritating tissue. And they layer. Cereal at breakfast, fruit juice at lunch, fast food at dinner. Each small exposure is a whisper the body hears as threat. Over time, those whispers swell.

Inside the gut, the lining works like a sieve that tightens with age. In infancy it's wide open by design, built to absorb antibodies from milk and messages from microbes. Research in both animal models and human populations suggests that certain modern additives may interfere with that maturation process, with some studies linking emulsifiers and highly processed food components to changes in gut barrier function. When the lining is compromised, fragments can slip into circulation, the immune system reads invasion and sounds the alarm, and the child shows what they can't explain: fatigue, tantrums, sleep fracturing for no visible reason. The science here is active and accumulating rather than settled, but the direction is consistent enough that parents tracking these patterns in their own children are watching something real.

The blood-brain barrier tells a related story. It's a living filter, cells joined by seals that tighten across early childhood. Research shows that sustained systemic inflammation, the kind that follows chronic immune activation, can affect barrier integrity and contribute to neurological symptoms in both children and adults. The precise mechanisms by which early dietary and environmental exposures drive this process in young children are still being worked out, and human longitudinal data is still accumulating. What's already established is the communication network itself: the gut, immune system, and brain share a chemical language, and disruption in one system sends signals the others respond to. Parents call it unpredictability. Science calls it cross-talk. Either way, the child endures it.

Individual biology shapes how much any of this matters for a given child. Some children's barriers are leakier by default, with genetic variants weakening linings and seals. Others inherit slower detox pathways or more reactive immune cells. What's benign to one child can ignite another. Biology doesn't obey averages, and that's precisely why population-level studies so often miss what parents living beside a specific nervous system can see.

The damage is rarely dramatic at first. The child still plays, laughs, grows, passes screenings, and smiles for photos. But erosion stacks underneath: membranes under pressure, circuits learning instability as normal. By the time symptoms surface, the nervous system has already been adapting to its conditions for months.

Most parents are taught to watch for fevers and hives, not to recognize that their child's body is still learning the difference between inside and out. They're taught to track milestones, not to understand that what touches their child's tongue can echo in their brain. They're taught to manage behavior, not to see that behavior can be biology's way of screaming.

It's easy to miss, because culture confuses growth with health. As long as height and weight climb, the details hide. But resilience is more than size. It's the ability to sleep without struggle, to stay calm under stress, and to learn without overload. When those capacities crumble, it's rarely random.

Modern childhood surrounds unfinished bodies with artificial inputs: foods that destabilize, air that irritates, light that overstimulates. The irony is cruel. A physiology built for steady signals now swims in noise.

The most haunting part is that the same inputs raising these concerns are marketed as care: fortified crackers, chewable vitamins. The world calls it nourishment. The body registers the mismatch. That gap fans a steady drift, a subtle shift in baseline tone. A child who never quite rests, who overreacts to texture, light, and sound. The body reads the world as a constant low-grade threat, and repair never fully catches up.

Parents often sense this drift before anyone else does. Something changes after lunch, they say. She's fine until the afternoon. That intuition is data that labs don't capture. You can't always see the disruption on a chart, but it reveals itself in rhythm.

Early inputs don't pass through children. They pass into

them. This is permeability. What enters a developing brain doesn't stay at the edges; it reaches circuitry still wiring itself. Each molecule leaves a mark, becoming part of the story the brain tells about the world.

Early years decide how loud the world will always sound. When you understand that a child's body is still building its walls, you start to see the cracks, and you seal where you can.

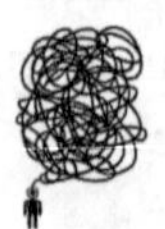

CHAPTER 14

CLARITY IS YOUR POWER

YOU DIDN'T BUILD this food system. You didn't approve the additives lining supermarket shelves or the school menus that pass for nutrition. You didn't write the guidelines that reduce health to calories and weight. Yet here you stand in the fallout, holding the child who absorbs its consequences.

That position is where your power begins.

For a long time, you doubted what you saw. Doubting felt safer than being wrong. Doctors called it a phase. Teachers called it growing pains. Friends said kids will be kids. You wanted to believe them because belief promised rest, and rest was something you hadn't had in months. But rest never came. Patterns did. The same meltdown after breakfast. The same fog after birthday parties. The same sleeplessness on nights that should've been ordinary. Once you started keeping track, something shifted. The confusion didn't deepen. It organized.

Clarity is the quiet after gaslight.

Every parent who arrives at this moment describes it the same way: a stillness that spreads through the chest, a stopping of the internal argument. The body recognizes what the mind had been working to dismiss. Fog lifts after steady meals. Rhythm returns as volatility recedes. The pattern that felt like

44

paranoia reveals itself as observation. Knowing steadies you in a way that reassurance never could, because reassurance required you to trust someone else's read over your own. Clarity requires only that you trust what you've already seen.

It centers you inside a large system. You stop swinging between advice and guilt and begin reading what's actually in front of you. When something helps, you note it. When something harms, you stop building explanations for why it shouldn't. You collect reality until it outweighs denial, and denial loses the quiet authority it once had over your choices.

This shift changes what you're looking for. The question becomes what does my child's biology say, rather than what do the guidelines say. Those two questions rarely produce the same answer, and now you know which one to trust. You learn which foods hold your child steady through an afternoon and which ones turn the hour after dinner into something you spend all day dreading. You learn which mornings begin with enough protein to carry a child through second period and which ones end in a call from the school before lunch. You learn the hours that matter and the rhythms that repair, and you learn them from watching the same body respond to the same inputs across enough days to be certain, rather than from a label or a handout.

Then something happens that most parents don't anticipate: the loneliness of this begins to ease. You find another parent who pulled dyes from the pantry and watched aggression follow them out. You find a father who added protein to breakfast and watched his daughter sit through homework for the first time in months. You find a mother who changed nothing but the dinner hour and got her child's sleep back. They're running the only experiment that matters: the one with their own child, tracked across their own kitchen, held against their own weeks of before and after. This is field research conducted in real time, and it accumulates into something the published literature rarely captures because no one funds it. The collective record of parents who stopped waiting for permission is one of the most reliable bodies of evidence available on how the modern food environment actually behaves inside a developing nervous system.

That record doesn't erase the cost of arriving here. Clarity's uncomfortable. Once you see the architecture of harm embedded in ordinary ritual, a birthday table becomes a different object. A school lunch tray becomes a different document. The ingredients in a fortified snack bar become a different kind of statement about what society has decided children are worth. Grief and relief arrive together in that moment, as they tend to when something long suspected is finally confirmed. Grief for the years spent trusting a system that was never designed with your child's biology in mind. Relief for finally understanding why the same inputs kept producing the same suffering.

Some parents move through that grief into anger, and anger has its uses. It names the betrayal clearly. But anger aimed at a faceless architecture is expensive fuel, and it burns through resources your child's biology actually needs from you: steadiness, presence, and the sustained attention required to keep changing what can be changed. The parents who hold their ground longest let the anger inform rather than consume. They remember what it cost not to see, and they use that memory as orientation rather than wound.

The work ahead is quieter than it sounds from the outside and largely unglamorous. It looks like cooking when you're exhausted. Like packing a lunch when the cafeteria would be easier. Like reading an ingredient list in a fluorescent aisle when everyone beside you is simply putting the box in the cart. It looks like saying no to the birthday cupcake and absorbing the social friction that follows, then watching your child hold their afternoon together in a way they couldn't the week before. It looks like doing this again tomorrow, and the day after, because consistency is the only language biology actually speaks. Perfection's not the goal.

There'll be days of compromise. There'll be weeks when the system wins more than you do, when the school lunch is what it is and the party food is everywhere and exhaustion makes the careful choice impossible. Those days aren't failure. They're the reality of operating inside a system you didn't design, with the resources you actually have. What changes with clarity isn't the difficulty of the work. What changes is that you no longer mistake a hard week for evidence that the work doesn't matter.

You're making different choices in the moments where different choices are possible, and watching those choices accumulate into a different trajectory. That's a form of power the system didn't intend for you to have.

Biology's still speaking, in every meal, every morning, every hour before bed. The difference now is that you're fluent, and fluency changes what's possible.

Do This Before Your Next Appointment

Swap one snack. Replace one refined snack (chips, cookies, soda...) with a whole-food choice. An apple. A string cheese. A boiled egg. Watch what steadiness feels like.

Keep a 2-day log. Write down what your child ate, when, and how their energy, mood, and focus shifted. Notice patterns that repeat—the body always leaves clues.

Use this script. "I've noticed energy dips about ninety minutes after certain foods. How can we track and test this further?"

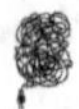

EVERY MOLECULE IS INSTRUCTION. When the instruction turns chaotic, biology signals for help, and when the signal grows loud enough, the system sends in a different kind of chemistry. Not to address what food did to the terrain, but to quiet what the terrain is saying.

When classrooms can't contain the volatility, pills promise focus. When sleep collapses, prescriptions promise rest. When moods swing wide, chemicals promise balance. Big Pharma arrives where Big Food left off, and the fire beneath keeps burning while the smoke gets managed.

Part Three asks what we lose when treatment outruns truth.

REFERENCES

1. Centers for Disease Control and Prevention. (2024, October 4). *About Chronic Diseases*. Retrieved from https://www.cdc.gov/chronic-disease/about/index.html

2. Chandler, A. (2019). *Drive-Thru Dreams: A Journey Through the Heart of America's Fast-Food Kingdom*. Flatiron Books. ISBN: 978-1250090720

3. Curtis, A. (2018). *Eat This!: How Fast-Food Marketing Gets You to Buy Junk (And How You Can Fight Back)*. Red Deer Press. ISBN: 978-0889955325

4. Fabbri, A., et al. (2018). Food industry sponsorship of academic research: Investigating commercial bias in the research agenda. *Public Health Nutrition, 21*(10), 1973–1981. https://doi.org/10.1017/S1368980018002100

5. Kearns, C. E., et al. (2016). Sugar industry and coronary heart disease research: A historical analysis of internal industry documents. *JAMA Internal Medicine*. https://doi.org/10.1001/jamainternmed.2016.5394

6. Mahase, E. (2023). US dietary committee is plagued with "high risk conflicts of interest," report finds. *BMJ, 383*, p2313. https://doi.org/10.1136/bmj.p2313

7. Moss, M. (2014). *Salt Sugar Fat: How the Food Giants Hooked Us*. Random House. ISBN: 978-0812982190

8. Nestle, M. (2007). *Food Politics: How the Food Industry Influences Nutrition and Health*. University of California Press. ISBN: 978-0520254039

9. Nestle, M. (2018). *Unsavory Truth: How Food Companies Skew the Science of What We Eat*. Basic Books. ISBN: 978-1541697119

10. Schlosser, E. (2001). *Fast Food Nation: The Dark Side of the All-American Meal*. Houghton Mifflin Harcourt. ISBN: 978-0547750330

11. Suez, J., et al. (2014). Artificial sweeteners induce glucose intolerance by altering the gut microbiota. *Nature*. https://doi.org/10.1038/nature13793

12. Van Tulleken, C. (2023). *Ultra-Processed People: The Science Behind Food That Isn't Food*. W.W. Norton & Company. ISBN: 978-1-324-07626-1

PART 3
BIG PHARMA

A SYSTEM, NOT A PRESCRIPTION

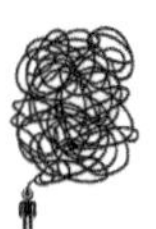

CHAPTER 15

RELIEF WITHOUT A WHY

THE STORY DOESN'T BEGIN in a lab or a boardroom. It begins in a child's body, where cells strain to keep pace with demands they were never meant to carry. Over time, capacity shifts. What once came easily — learning, patience, recovery — starts to take genuine effort, and to the outside world it looks like ordinary childhood turbulence: a bad week, a stubborn phase, a growth spurt expected to pass. But inside, the balance between stress and restoration is already tilting. Injury stacks faster than the body can clear it, and repair falls further behind.

That's where Big Pharma enters. A parent brings a story, and what was once a living rhythm gets reduced to a symptom list. The search for cause turns into a race for control, and then the prescription appears. Physiology is recast as pharmacology.

Picture a child who can't sit still: legs in motion, pencil tapping, gaze darting as if stillness burns. Or a child who cries every morning before school, gripping the doorway as though their body knows what their words can't yet say. Maybe they're six and already whispering that they hate themselves, or nine, sitting under fluorescent lights with an IEP longer than their moments of true learning. In that swirl of frustration, fatigue, and fear, a lifeline appears. It arrives as a practiced phrase, spoken in a calm clinical tone: "There's a medication that might help."

You want that to be true. It sounds reasonable and compassionate, and medicine is supposed to ease suffering. What parent would refuse relief when their child is hurting? The room shifts, shoulders drop, and promise enters the air. In that moment, asking for more feels reckless.

One father pressed anyway. He asked what could be driving his son's daily aggression, and the physician paused long enough to order a sleep study before writing anything. It showed severe fragmentation with insufficient slow-wave sleep, despite the child being in bed all night. There was no apnea and no seizure activity, only chronic under-recovery. Circadian timing, evening light exposure, and daytime sleep pressure were corrected first. Within weeks, the aggression had softened by half, and with the system no longer in free fall, medication was introduced at a small dose. Side effects were avoided, and the child woke calm. That wasn't an exception.

Another parent pressed differently. After her son began an anxiety medication that left him wired through the night, she asked a simple question: what happens in his brain while he sleeps? They checked ferritin rather than hemoglobin alone, because iron stores shape dopamine tone and night arousal. His ferritin was low. Iron was repleted, and bedtime was rebuilt with dim lights, an earlier dinner, and a protected final hour free of blue light and noise. As sleep deepened, the dose that had once made him edgy began to actually help. Answers rarely come without questions.

Parents often hear words that sound clinical and land like verdicts: chemical imbalance, neurodevelopmental disorder. They're told that without medication things may worsen and windows will close, and it's implied that any hesitation is the wrong choice. The script is framed as the ethical path. What rarely gets said is this: symptoms don't appear from nowhere. They're provoked by ultra-processed diets that destabilize fuel and flood synapses with noise, by environments that demand stillness while punishing movement, by chronic stress that warps cortisol rhythms and traps the nervous system in survival mode, and by broken sleep that denies neurons their nightly reset. For children whose genes already tilt toward fragility, these pressures are accelerants. The exam room isn't built to hold that whole picture. Time is short and stories are long. Tests that reveal nuance aren't prioritized, and the work of restoring terrain takes time that the system rarely allocates. Rather than asking why a child is struggling, the system more often asks how quickly the struggle can be silenced. Speed becomes the measure, and silence becomes the proof.

But silence can mean two very different things. It can mean a signal has been decoded and its driver removed, the body exhaling because demand finally meets supply. Or it can mean the signal has been suppressed while load keeps rising underneath. To a busy classroom and a tired family, both can look like success, but only one is repair.

There's a way to tell which one you're holding: look for depth. When relief is real, it carries across settings. It shows up in the morning and holds through the afternoon. Sleep arrives without chemical force, curiosity appears without coaxing, transitions ease, and play returns. Appetite steadies, and the nervous system recovers after stress rather than shattering from it. When relief is only surface, compliance carries a cost. Appetite thins, sleep fragments, evenings erupt as doses fade, and quiet collapses under real load.

None of this makes medication the enemy. The right drug in the right context can lift a child out of a choke point they can't climb alone. It can quiet panic and keep a family safe. The question isn't whether relief is allowed. It's whether relief is aligned.

Aligned relief sits on protected ground. It comes after sleep is guarded, fuel steadied, and movement woven into the day. It arrives with a plan for the smallest effective dose and the slowest possible rise. It honors how developing brains respond to change and measures benefit and harm together, in the same accounting, on review dates set before the first pill is swallowed. Misaligned relief rushes. It treats the symptom as the problem and the body as background, asking a miswired brain to carry more for the sake of quiet. Short-term quiet can mask long-term cost, and relief that ignores cause is delay dressed as care.

You can consent to treatment without surrendering the question, or the criteria that govern it. You see the patterns and you know whether things hold or fall apart when the pressure is real. You live the aftermath. You get to ask why.

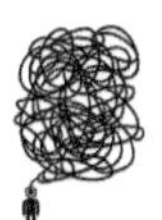

CHAPTER 16

SPEED ISN'T HEALING

FEW INSTITUTIONS HAVE SAVED MORE lives than the pharmaceutical industry. Antibiotics ended infections that once killed without mercy. Insulin turned a death sentence into a manageable condition. Antiepileptics shielded brains from repeated electrical storms. These are real triumphs, earned and consequential and undeniable. Alongside them runs another, less visible story: an industry that learned to monetize urgency, that learned how fear accelerates demand, and that learned to confuse speed with healing. In that story, the child in front of you shifts from a body under strain to a noise to quiet quickly.

Modern pharmaceuticals were forged in industrial chemistry. In the late nineteenth century, German dye manufacturers discovered that coal-tar chemistry could produce drugs as well as color, and companies like Bayer and BASF grew from pigment to pill. Wartime accelerated production of stimulants and sedatives for soldiers, and after the wars, those same manufacturing systems were repurposed for civilian consumption. In the United States, companies like Merck, Pfizer, and Lilly translated wartime chemistry into peacetime markets. From the beginning, urgency and chemistry moved together as these companies chased bigger profits. The breakthroughs were dazzling, but ambition often outran caution. Repeated and widespread safety disasters prompted new regulations, and growth kept outpacing restraint.

By the late 1990s, when direct-to-consumer advertising was legalized in the United States, the boundary between clinic and culture dissolved. Commercials entered living rooms and trumpeted medication benefits with borrowed authority, and the message repeated until it felt clinical: ask your doctor. Culture shifted with it. Streaming erased pauses. E-commerce collapsed delay into a click. Notifications trained nervous systems to expect immediate confirmation, and immediacy began to feel like competence. That conditioning made waiting feel like failure. Parents didn't want to wait months for therapy access. Schools couldn't absorb prolonged disruption. Physicians didn't want to feel ineffective. And Big Pharma offered an answer that promised relief now.

Stimulants became the emblem of that promise. A restless child could appear calmer within days. Teachers relaxed, parents exhaled, and charts improved. The speed was seductive and the relief felt decisive. The calm was visible. The strain wasn't.

A ten-year-old boy named Isaac began medication after months of classroom chaos. Within a week, his teacher wrote home: "A new child!" Homework was finished, the calls stopped, and the family finally slept. Two months later, the costs surfaced. He couldn't fall asleep before midnight, his appetite thinned, his skin paled, and he chewed through the collar of every shirt. When the medication wore off, his aggression returned sharper than before. What was labeled "wearing off" was depletion. The same chemistry that quieted his behavior increased metabolic demand in his body, pushing energy requirements beyond what his developing brain could sustain. This is how speed misleads. It delivers visible change before the invisible costs are counted. Suppression passes for stability because it's fast.

Repair requires something different: fuel that steadies, sleep that restores, and enough time for stress to metabolize. Clinical trials aren't built to capture that distinction. They're measured in weeks rather than years, and six weeks of symptom reduction becomes success even though developing brains don't heal on trial timelines. They build, prune, and adapt over long arcs, with resilience emerging through cycles of nourishment and rest. Markets run on clocks. Biology doesn't.

That mismatch shapes the entire research ecosystem. When drug development adopts the market's tempo, curiosity becomes the first casualty. Questions about what preceded the symptom, how terrain shaped response, or what timing reveals about cumulative load all slow momentum and threaten returns. Trials stay short because capital demands speed. Journals reward novelty over durability. The metric becomes rate of reduction rather than strength of restoration. It's like judging a seed by how quickly it sprouts rather than whether it survives the season.

Inside this tempo, caution starts to look irresponsible. Parents who want to stabilize context before starting medication are labeled resistant. Physicians who suggest slower titration are seen as outdated. Schools count days until quiet and call that progress. Patience is reframed as negligence. But biology keeps its own cadence. Energy doesn't rush its cycles. The nervous system recalibrates in rhythm with light, rest, and safety. Neuroplasticity unfolds in waves rather than leaps, and resilience takes time. Shorten that time, and you interrupt the very processes meant to protect the child. Speed looks like action and sounds like compassion and reads like progress, but it flattens nuance and confuses motion with direction. What it buys in weeks, it often extracts in endurance.

Some families learn this painfully. One mother told me, "We gained quiet but lost him." Her son's anxiety medication erased panic and dimmed the light that made him curious. His drawings stopped and his laughter faded. He wasn't suffering the same way, but he wasn't himself either. It was only when the pace slowed, sleep was protected, diet adjusted, and the dose carefully reduced that his light returned. It took seven months, but it held.

That's the paradox at the center of this chapter: what's built fast breaks fast. Speed isn't healing.

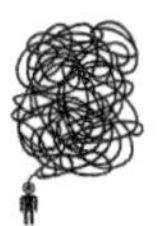

CHAPTER 17

FROM RELIEF TO RELIANCE

WHAT BEGAN as relief becomes maintenance, and what began as safety becomes dependency. The shift is rarely dramatic.

A medication produces a change. The chart looks better and symptoms ease just enough to declare success. From there, the measure mutates. Treatment is no longer judged by whether the body recovers, but by whether the result holds. Relief becomes something to preserve, and preservation demands consistency. Consistency becomes repetition, and repetition breeds tolerance. Receptors adapt. Signaling pathways adjust. What worked yesterday works less today, and the dose that helped becomes the dose that helped then. To restore the effect, the amount rises.

This is dose creep. It always arrives as a small adjustment: a fraction more, a timing change, a second daily dose to smooth the edge. Each is justified in isolation. Together, they reset the baseline.

Side effects appear next, framed as tradeoffs. An appetite suppressant for weight gain, a sleep aid for insomnia, a mood stabilizer for irritability that wasn't there before. Each addition is framed as necessary care, and stacking becomes normal. The system interprets this accumulation as optimization rather than escalation. Each prescription has a target, each target has an urgency, and the body fades from view as its parts are treated separately.

With time, the reference point moves. What once would have been flagged is now expected, and what once would have raised concern is now routine. Language shifts to accommodate permanence: "This is how they do on it." "This is as good as it gets." "This is stable."

Attempts to reduce are sometimes haphazard. Withdrawal effects follow, mislabeled as relapse, and the system responds by restoring the dose or adding another agent to control the reaction. The original question, whether the body is actually recovering, disappears from consideration. Exit becomes risky. Maintenance becomes the goal.

At this stage, the child's physiology is no longer the primary variable. The regimen is. Decisions are made in the name of stability rather than capacity, and the system stops asking what the body needs and reorganizes instead around maintaining what's already prescribed. Doses rise. Combinations grow.

This is reliance. It doesn't require bad intent, and it doesn't require error. It requires only tolerance and time.

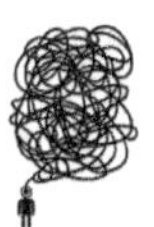

CHAPTER 18

BRIDGES, NOT SCAFFOLDS

THIS ISN'T a condemnation of medication. Some drugs save lives outright, and that's beyond dispute. Antibiotics stop sepsis. Insulin keeps children alive. Antiepileptics prevent repeated injury. These interventions continue to matter. But alongside those triumphs runs a structural failure. The pharmaceutical industry's original mandate was to preserve function and reduce suffering during acute threat, and over time that mandate drifted. Tools designed for short-term stabilization became instruments of long-term management. What should have served as bridges hardened into permanent scaffolds.

Parents feel that drift in the exam room. Your teen can't sleep, can't sit still, or can't stop crying. You bring your data: meltdowns after meals, panic at transitions. The physician listens, nods, and prescribes, with action dressed as compassion. The frame narrows quickly. The brain is struggling, and the fix is pharmacologic.

Antidepressants reveal the risk of that narrowing. SSRIs are prescribed to children and adolescents for anxiety and depression even though the trials behind them were brief and conducted largely in adults. Meanwhile, a child's serotonin system is still forming, shaped by nutrition, sleep, stress, and developmental timing. Altering that system during development isn't a neutral act. It reshapes physiology while physiology is still being built. Emotional flattening, weight changes, and paradoxical agitation are well documented, and long-term outcomes remain uncertain because few studies follow children across decades. Prescriptions are written anyway.

A twelve-year-old girl I met had been started on an SSRI after eight weeks of relentless worry. Her appetite dulled and her sparkle dimmed, but her test scores eventually improved. They called it progress.

Stimulants follow the same pattern, just faster. Methylphenidate and amphetamine salts can transform outward behavior almost overnight, flooding attention circuits with dopamine and norepinephrine, sharpening focus while increasing metabolic demand. Appetite suppression destabilizes fuel as sleep fragments, and the child may look regulated while living on a physiological edge, with chemistry replacing capacity. The story behind this isn't new. In the 1990s, stimulants once marketed to soldiers and secretaries were repackaged for children, with restlessness reframed as a chronic disorder. Marketing sold the idea that stillness could be manufactured, and sales exploded.

Antipsychotics darken the trajectory further. Developed for severe psychiatric illness, they're now prescribed to children for tantrums and irritability. Some uses are approved, but many aren't, and the side effects can be profound, with metabolic injury and movement disorders among them. Dopamine fuels curiosity and motivation, and when it's blunted, tantrums may fade while vitality fades with them. Parents often describe a flatter, less engaged child. The system calls it treatment.

Medication is meant to return children to a state where repair is possible. Too often, it suppresses symptoms while the body remains unstable underneath, managing without mending.

A true pharmacologic bridge supports repair. Consider June, a seven-year-old with severe tics who was given a low-dose antiepileptic for five months while sleep and magnesium were intentionally restored. Inhibition pathways recovered as the drug quieted sensory overload, and when the dose tapered, the tics stayed gone. Repair ensured that she could hold the gain.

A scaffold looks different. Prescriptions stack as side effects appear: appetite drugs for stimulant weight loss, sleep drugs for stimulant insomnia, mood drugs for stimulant rebound. Soon, no one remembers which pill began the climb. Chemistry accumulates until the regimen, rather than the child, becomes the point of reference.

Bridges shorten dependency. Scaffolds extend it. Bridges are planned with exits. Scaffolds are maintained with fear. If a drug creates space for repair, it's a bridge. If it replaces repair, it's a scaffold.

None of this means medication is a betrayal. It means bridge, not scaffold.

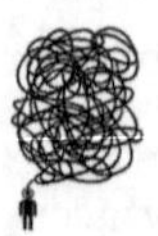

CHAPTER 19
ASK QUESTIONS

BY THE TIME most families face the question of whether to medicate, they aren't arriving fresh. They're scraped and worn thin. They've fielded calls that land like alarms, held a shaking child through midnight panic, and absorbed the stares of strangers who treat collapse as a character flaw. Inside, guilt wrestles exhaustion while hope wrestles despair. When the offer comes, it feels like a lifeline. Some parents say yes immediately. Some wait until fatigue breaks resolve. Some say no and guard what little ground feels stable. None of these choices are moral verdicts. They're decisions made inside scarcity: of sleep, of time, of clarity.

A prescription carries weight far beyond the screen it's entered on. To a desperate parent, it feels like an answer, finally. You want something that works. You want your child out of pain. You want reprieve. So when the question comes, medicate or not, it carries the full weight of what it means to be a good parent. But what if that isn't the right question? What if that frame skips what actually matters?

Diagnosis isn't the plot. Medication isn't the main character. The better question is more precise: what is this symptom trying to say?

Children don't erupt, withdraw, or shut down at random. They're adaptive organisms, not broken machines, and symptoms are the nervous system speaking, the body metabolizing load in the only language it has. Every outburst, refusal, or collapse is a translation of distress. When we learn to read those signals, the story changes. We stop treating survival instinct as pathology. We stop reading explosions as proof of brokenness and start asking what lit the fuse. We notice whether meals destabilize fuel, whether nights fracture repair, or whether stress accumulates without release. We ask whether genetic vulnerability thins resilience, whether mitochondrial strain, redox imbalance, or immune priming shapes the day. What looks like defiance may be erratic supply. What looks like withdrawal may be preservation of last reserves.

Big Pharma trains us to ask a narrower question: what label fits? Distress gets medicated before it's decoded, and the asking stops there. The deeper question is whether we're listening closely enough to know what the distress is actually asking for.

The deepest wound forms in identity, in the child who absorbs a message we never intend them to learn: your body is the problem. The better message is already there, waiting to be spoken: your body is speaking. Let's learn to listen.

Medication can play a supportive role. Sometimes it buys time. Sometimes it keeps a child safe. Sometimes it opens a window wide enough for learning to return. But it shouldn't be the only tool, and it shouldn't move forward without asking what's driving the storm.

So how do you discern? How do you tell when a drug supports healing and when it only buys quiet?

Start by refusing to be rushed. Pause, and then ask what you're treating, exactly, and how you'll measure it. Name one primary target and a timeframe. Fewer panic jolts at bedtime over four weeks. Less afternoon classroom removals. Specificity prevents drift.

Ask what medical checks come first. Rule out the drivers that mimic or magnify symptoms: iron status, thyroid function, sleep apnea, seizures, medication side effects, unstable fuel supply. Clarity before chemistry.

Ask what supports begin now, and who owns them. Sleep structure, protein and mineral intake, outdoor movement, sensory supports, stress offload. Assign names and dates, because ownership creates follow-through.

If you start medication, go in with a plan. Begin with the lowest dose, titrate slowly, review weekly, and track benefit and harm together. Decide in advance what counts as working, because slow titration protects the developing brain in ways that speed cannot.

Ask about the course and the exit before the first dose is swallowed. Set duration, review dates, and exit criteria. If the body stabilizes, outline a taper. Every beginning deserves a planned ending.

Ask what's known and what remains unknown: short-term effects, interactions, withdrawal risks, and the limits of long-term data in developing brains. Uncertainty acknowledged is harm reduced.

And keep asking, through every phase: Is sleep full? Is fuel steady? Is stress being metabolized? Are sensory needs honored? Is movement built into the day? Are signs of cumulative disruption being addressed? These aren't optional additions to the plan. Everything else depends on them, and they're the first things sacrificed to speed while medication moves forward without meaning.

A system without consequence will always cut corners. Ask questions.

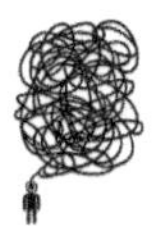

CHAPTER 20

PILLS FALL SHORT

MODERN MEDICINE PROMISES PRECISION. Pills are marketed as targeted, molecules framed as elegant solutions, and the language suggests finesse, control, and mastery. But biology isn't impressed by precision that ignores context.

A drug can alter signaling. It can dampen output and quiet a body under strain. What it often can't do is rebuild the biology that made collapse likely in the first place. It can't create sleep where sleep feels unsafe. It can't stabilize fuel where supply spikes and crashes. It can't metabolize stress that never resolves. A pill can lower the volume, but it can't change the song.

This is the limit drug companies rarely name.

Most pharmaceuticals are designed to act on biology rather than to supply what a child's body actually needs in order to repair. They intervene downstream, after demand has already outrun capacity, and when they work, they often do so by suppressing signals that were never the problem, only the messenger. The illusion is control: the belief that a molecule can override a nervous system still operating inside instability, that output can be corrected without addressing the conditions driving the strain.

Most nervous systems don't fail because a molecule is missing. They fail because repair can't keep pace with demand. Pills can't make a body feel safe enough to heal, and they can't create the rhythms that development depends on. This doesn't make medication useless. It makes it incomplete.

Incompleteness is rarely acknowledged, because acknowledging it would require admitting what pharmaceuticals aren't designed to address and widening the lens beyond what a molecule can correct. Instead, medication becomes the stand-in for the protection that modern life won't provide. Pills arrive faster than food systems can be repaired, faster than stress can be metabolized, faster than childhood can unfold. And because the intervention is visible, it feels sufficient. But medication conceals the fallout rather than correcting what caused it.

Once symptom control is mistaken for repair, signals get ignored. Progress is declared while capacity continues to erode, and the system moves on. Evidence narrows from there. The system decides which outcomes qualify as evidence and which costs vanish from view. What resolves quickly is counted. What unfolds slowly disappears.

Why do pills fall short? Look upstream.

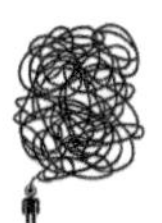

CHAPTER 21

WHEN SCIENCE GETS CURATED

WE WANT to believe science is a fortress, that data are clean, that journals are neutral, and that experts stand guard immune to persuasion. Parents cling to that hope because if it isn't true, then trust feels like sand. But drugs don't live in a vacuum. They live inside an ecosystem, and that ecosystem is profitable.

The pharmaceutical industry didn't just learn how to make drugs. It learned how to shape how those drugs are understood, taught, and defended. Start with Continuing Medical Education, the training that keeps licenses active. You imagine your child's doctor learning unbiased advances. In reality, much of it is underwritten by the same companies whose products are being taught. The funding doesn't always dictate the words on a slide, but it narrows the field. It selects the topics, chooses the messengers, and rewards certain conclusions with more airtime.

Regulation carries its own pressure. Fast-track pathways can accelerate access for people who truly need new treatments, and they can also accelerate profit. Industry and regulators often share personnel, language, and incentives. Patents are extended through new formulations and small pivots that stretch revenue long after discovery. Insurers reinforce the pattern by reimbursing what's easiest to code. The pill fits the system. The upstream work rarely does.

Publishing echoes the same structure. Many journals rely on advertising and sponsorship to survive, and some studies are designed, drafted, and even ghostwritten with industry involvement. When findings don't favor the funder, they may be delayed, reframed, or never published at all. When they do favor the funder, they're amplified. Reviews and meta-analyses pool what's visible and call it consensus, and clinical guidelines then crystallize that consensus into standard of care, often written by committees with undisclosed financial ties.

Advocacy can become another filter. Parent foundations and awareness campaigns are often born from real pain and real love, but many are funded in part by the same corporations that manufacture the treatments they promote. Language shifts over time. A condition once described with nuance becomes framed as inevitably lifelong. Hesitation becomes stigma. Questions become denial. The result isn't always better health. Sometimes it's a larger market and a narrower imagination.

That isn't a conspiracy. There's no secret plot, no smoking-gun bribe, no villain twirling a mustache, no doctor knowingly lying to you, and no scientist falsifying data in a dark room. It's ordinary people operating inside a system whose incentives bend outcomes, incentives doing what incentives do. Most clinicians believe they're acting ethically. Most researchers follow the rules in front of them. But when funding, publication, promotion, and reimbursement all reward the same narrow kind of answer, the system drifts without anyone having to be the bad actor.

Blind to this machinery, you walk into the exam room believing recommendations rise from neutral evidence. You don't see the sponsored symposium that shaped the talking points, the honorarium, the glossy sample packs, or the collaboration email. You see a white coat and you hope. This is how science gets curated: by selection and by filters. What gets funded determines what gets asked. What gets published determines what gets taught. What gets taught determines what gets prescribed.

You can see the downstream consequence in a single sentence: "Studies show it's safe." Often, the pediatrician is simply repeating what the pipeline curated. But safe may have been defined by eight-week trials using endpoints that capture symptom change while missing developmental cost. The statement can be technically true and still incomplete.

None of this erases the breakthroughs that changed the world. Antibiotics still save lives. Insulin still sustains them. Antiepileptics still guard neurons. But the same pipeline that delivered those miracles can also filter reality through economics, bias, and the modern attention span. Families stand at the end of that pipeline, trying to make decisions with partial light. Asking where the light came from isn't paranoia. It's responsibility.

Transparency shouldn't threaten science. It should strengthen it. Funding sources should be declared, data should be shared, and conflicts should be named aloud. Trust grows sturdier that way, and parents can handle complexity. Prudence doesn't mean rejecting science. It means demanding its full story. Who funded this? What got excluded? What happens long term in a developing brain?

It also means noticing what isn't studied. There's robust data on antidepressant molecules, particularly in adults, and far less on how sleep debt, circadian disruption, micronutrient depletion, or unstable fuel supply reshape neurotransmission in children over time. Because no one owns the patent on darkness, or protein, or a regulated nervous system. What can't be monetized gets underfunded, what's underfunded looks unproven, and what looks unproven gets ignored.

The exam room isn't insulated from influence. It lives and

breathes it. The counterweight strong enough to steady the frame is informed, calm discernment. Truth doesn't need purity to stand. It needs light.

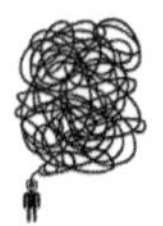

CHAPTER 22

COMPLIANCE ISN'T DEVELOPMENT

WE'VE BEEN TAUGHT to measure children by behavior. A quiet classroom. A finished worksheet. A school day that ends without a call home. When the disruptions stop and homework gets done without tears, relief feels like progress and looks like proof. The chart improves. The teacher relaxes. The family exhales. Everyone agrees it's working.

But the question worth asking is what, exactly, is working.

A child isn't thriving simply because the screaming stopped. Silence has more than one cause, and stillness has more than one meaning. Sometimes a quiet child is a regulated child, one whose nervous system has genuinely found its footing, whose body is resting inside a window of real stability. That's the outcome worth working toward. But sometimes quiet is exhaustion wearing a familiar face. Sometimes it's suppression, a nervous system conserving what little energy remains rather than expressing what it feels. Sometimes it's a child who's learned that the cost of showing distress is higher than the cost of absorbing it, and who's made the calculation so many times it's become automatic. From the outside, these look identical. The chart captures behavior. It doesn't capture mechanism.

This is where the compliance standard breaks down, because compliance is a performance metric and development is a biological one, and those two things don't always move in the same direction. A child can comply completely while developing poorly. A child can hold it together through every school hour and spend the evening paying back the cost of that effort in ways no checklist records: meltdowns after pickup, food refusal at dinner, sleep that won't arrive, a body that can't come down from the vigilance it's been maintaining all day. The performance was real. The recovery cost was real. The system counted the first and missed the second entirely.

Development doesn't unfold to please systems. It unfolds according to its own biological logic, which is indifferent to report cards and IEP goals and the preferences of a classroom schedule. When a brain shifts out of survival and back toward genuine growth, it often looks less tidy at first, not worse but wilder. More movement. More emotion. More friction at the edges of demands that once produced compliance without complaint. A child coming back online after a period of suppression may look, to the untrained eye, like a child getting worse. What's actually happening is that the nervous system is testing whether it's safe to express what it's been holding, and that testing takes up space that compliance had previously vacated.

Biology rarely reorganizes on command, and it rarely reorganizes quietly. What matters isn't how pliable a child becomes inside a given set of expectations. What matters is whether the body underneath those expectations is building capacity or spending it, accumulating resilience or running it down. Those are different trajectories, and they lead to different futures, and the compliance standard can't tell them apart because it was never designed to look that deep.

A nervous system held together by suppression is structurally fragile. It works while control is enforced, while the environment stays predictable, while the dose holds, while the demands stay within a range the child has learned to manage through effort rather than through genuine regulation. When any of those conditions shift, the structure reveals itself. Stress spikes and the child who seemed so improved shatters in ways that feel disproportionate because the baseline was never as solid as the behavior suggested. The stability was real but narrow, purchased through suppression rather than built through recovery, and suppression has carrying costs that compound quietly until they can't be hidden.

A nervous system rebuilt with adequate supply and genuine recovery is different in kind, not just degree. It restores itself after stress rather than fracturing under it. It absorbs disruption without losing its footing. It holds across settings, across times of day, across the unpredictable demands of an ordinary childhood, because its stability isn't borrowed from a shrinking reserve. It's generated from a system that's actually been replenished. That child can handle a hard afternoon without unraveling the evening. That child can miss a dose without a crisis. That child's calm travels with them rather than depending on conditions being exactly right.

The distance between those two children is invisible to the compliance standard. Both might score the same on a behavior rating scale. Both might produce the same teacher feedback. Both might sit in the same seat, produce the same worksheet, and exit the building at the same bell. The difference lives in the biology underneath the behavior, in whether the nervous system is spending or restoring, contracting or expanding, adapting toward resilience or adapting toward endurance. Systems reward compliance because it's visible, billable, and fast. Biology demands coherence because it's real, because a developing brain is building its architecture from the conditions it actually lives inside, and that architecture will outlast every metric used to assess it.

This is the cost of mistaking suppression for stability and

performance for health. It's a cost paid slowly, in the currency of developmental time, and it often doesn't surface until the child is older and the window for certain kinds of repair has narrowed. By then, the compliance has long since been credited as success, and the bill arrives without an obvious connection to the choices that generated it.

Parents often feel this mismatch before they can name it. They watch a child who by every external measure is doing better, and they feel something's still off. The laughter's a little thin. The eyes don't quite track the same way. The child who used to initiate play now waits to be told what to do. These are signals. They're the nervous system communicating in the register that compliance standards aren't built to hear, the register of aliveness rather than manageability, of genuine presence rather than behavioral output.

Children aren't meant to perform wellness. They're meant to experience it, to inhabit their own days from the inside rather than managing the appearance of those days for an audience of adults with clipboards. The goal of any real intervention, whether that's medication, therapy, nutritional change, or sleep restoration, is to create conditions where a child can develop rather than conditions where a child can comply. Those conditions look different and feel different and sometimes produce more friction in the short term because development is inherently dynamic and compliance is inherently static.

When the question shifts from is this child behaving to is this child building, everything downstream of that question changes. The metrics change. The timeline changes. The definition of success changes. A child who's noisier but more genuinely present becomes legible as progress rather than regression. A child who's pushing back against demands that once produced silent compliance becomes readable as a nervous system testing its newfound capacity rather than a treatment that's stopped working.

That shift in question is the one Big Pharma's model resists most, because a child who's genuinely developing needs less management over time, and less management is a different business outcome than the one the system is structured to produce. Compliance is a renewable market. Development is the goal that makes itself obsolete.

Ask for development. Settle for nothing less.

Do This Before Your Next Appointment

Name three behaviors. Write your child's three most improved symptoms since starting any intervention.

Ask the grounding question. For each, note: "Is this relief built on stability or suppression?"

Use this script. "I'm seeing improvement, but I'd like to understand what's driving it. Is this a sign of healing or a sign of silence?"

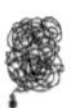

BEHIND EVERY PILL is a system that decided what care is allowed to look like, which symptoms deserve urgency, and which questions never get asked. That system is Big Medicine, and it shapes the exam room long before a family walks through the door.

A system built to heal began optimizing for billing and defensibility, and somewhere in that shift, diagnostic certainty overtook biological curiosity. The diagnosis now arrives before the question. Part Four traces how.

REFERENCES

1. Anderson, S. (2005). *Making Medicines: A Brief History of Pharmacy and Pharmaceuticals*. Pharmaceutical Press. ISBN: 978-0857110992.

2. Angell, M. (2005). *The Truth About the Drug Companies: How They Deceive Us and What to Do About It*. Random House. ISBN: 978-0375508462.

3. Ballentine, C. (1981). The Sulfanilamide Disaster. Retrieved from https://www.fda.gov/files/about%20fda/published/The-Sulfanil amide-Disaster.pdf.

4. Buratovich, M. (2022). Elixir Sulfanilamide Scandal. Retrieved from https://www.ebsco.com/research-starters/history/elixir-sulfanil amide-scandal.

5. Eban, K. (2019). *Bottle of Lies: The Inside Story of the Generic Drug Boom*. Ecco. ISBN: 978-0062338792.

6. Goldacre, B. (2013). *Bad Pharma: How Drug Companies Mislead Doctors and Harm Patients*. Faber & Faber. ISBN: 978-0865478008.

7. Gotzsche, P. (2013). *Deadly Medicines and Organised Crime* (1st Ed.). Radcliffe Publishing. ISBN: 978-1846198847.

8. Gross, D., & Sampat, B. (2025). The Therapeutic Consequences of the War: World War II and the 20th-Century Expansion of Biomedicine. Retrieved from https://www.nber.org/papers/w33457.

9. Healy, D. (2006). *Let Them Eat Prozac: The Unhealthy Relationship Between the Pharmaceutical Industry and Depression*. New York University Press. ISBN: 978-0814736975.

10. Kirsch, I. (2010). *The Emperor's New Drugs: Exploding the Antidepressant Myth*. Basic Books. ISBN: 978-0465022007.

11. Kirsch, I. (2019). Placebo Effect in the Treatment of Depression and Anxiety. Retrieved from https://pmc.ncbi.nlm.nih.gov/articles/PMC6584108/.

12. Miller, S.P. (2024). Germ theory of disease. *EBSCO Research Starters*. Retrieved from https://www.ebsco.com/research-starters/biology/germ-theory-disease.

13. Moynihan, R., & Cassels, A. (2005). *Selling Sickness: How the World's Biggest Pharmaceutical Companies Are Turning Us All Into Patients*. Nation Books. ISBN: 978-1560258568.

14. Petruzzello, M. (2023). Pure Food and Drug Act. *Encyclopedia Britannica*. Retrieved from https://www.britannica.com/topic/Pure-Food-and-Drug-Act.

15. Ross, J., & Krazitz, R. (2013). Direct-to-Consumer Television Advertising: Time to Turn Off the Tube? Retrieved from https://pmc.ncbi.nlm.nih.gov/articles/PMC3682047/.

16. Sismondo, S. (2018). *Ghost-Managed Medicine: Big Pharma's Invisible Hands*. Mattering Press. ISBN: 978-0995527775.

17. Tobbell, D. (2011). *Pills, Power, and Policy: The Struggle for Drug Reform in Cold War America and Its Consequences*. University of California Press. ISBN: 978-0520271142.

18. UMass Diabetes Center of Excellence. (2024). Banting & Best: The Discovery of Insulin. Retrieved from https://www.umassmed.edu/dcoe/diabetes-education/patient-resources/banting-and-best-discover-insulin.

19. Vanderbes, J. (2023). *Wonder Drug: The Secret History of Thalidomide in America and Its Hidden Victims*. Random House. ISBN: 978-0525512264.

20. Weatherall, M. (1990). *In Search of a Cure: A History of Pharmaceutical Discovery*. Oxford University Press. ISBN: 978-0192617477.

PART 4
BIG MEDICINE

A SYSTEM, NOT A VISIT

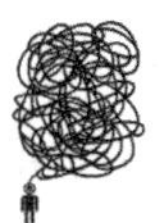

CHAPTER 23

THE MINUTE THAT MATTERS

IT'S 8:52 a.m. when they're finally called in. The printer hums. The cartoon loops on the wall. The toddler's eyes glaze from waiting-room screen time. The baby fusses in the car seat, feet kicking the blanket loose. She doesn't check her watch because she already knows the rhythm of this place. Diaper bag on one arm, car seat on the other, the older child trailing a bent-eared bunny that drags softly along the hall tile.

The medical assistant measures twenty-seven pounds and types it in, keys clicking faster than the words can land.

"Any fever?" "No, but he hasn't been himself." "Medications?" "No." "Allergies?" "No."

A pulse-ox cuff kisses a finger and beeps. "Okay, the doctor will be right in." The room is cold in that particular way clinics keep cold. The toddler whines. She opens crackers, wipes a nose, and rocks the car seat with her foot. In her mind, she rehearses the thing that matters. It isn't the sniffle, or whatever phone triage named last night. He used to say mama. Now there's nothing, and he doesn't turn to his name. The unease in her chest keeps its steady beat.

A knock. The pediatrician enters with a practiced smile, eyes already on the tablet. "Looks like we're here for a runny nose?"

She shakes her head, finds her place, and begins. "Actually, that's not why I . . ." He lifts the stethoscope. "Let's listen first." Chest. Lungs. Heart. The loop of motions he could do in his sleep. Everything sounds good. Probably a virus. Fluids and rest. Anything else?

Here it is. The moment she's rehearsed since his first word went missing. But the tempo is too fast and the air too thin. The visit's already ending. "I've noticed some changes," she says. "He used to talk a little. Now he doesn't say anything. He doesn't respond to his name." The doctor nods, smile held tight. Wide range of normal, especially for boys. Probably a phase. Let's keep an eye on it.

She swallows the rest. What she wants to say is this: he isn't in a phase. Please see it. Please help her name it. He turns to the tablet. Clicks quicken. Orders finalize. Windows close. Eleven minutes. That's all it lasted. What goes unsaid here will script the next two years.

9:03 a.m. Another mother, in another room, refuses the fade. She doesn't raise her voice, but she makes one thing non-negotiable: "I need to understand why my daughter wakes at 3 a.m. every night." The pediatrician pauses. The sentence lands like a weight. He orders a ferritin level he hadn't before considered, and it comes back low. With iron, sleep steadies. The child wakes to mornings that don't feel like glass. Her persistence shifts the arc.

9:17 a.m. A father arrives with three short videos. His son's eyes flick up, then his head dips. The clips look like nothing if you watch only a moment, so he asks the doctor to watch all the way through. Twenty seconds in, the pattern emerges: clusters, brief spells, subtle and easy to miss. The pediatrician orders an EEG, treatment begins, and language returns in small steps. For vulnerable wiring, that's how fast attention can change the brain's path.

9:41 a.m. A grandmother opens a notebook with meals on the left and what follows on the right, arrows drawn between them:

pasta to midnight screaming, red yogurt to hives. She doesn't use the words glycemic load or histamine, and she doesn't need them for the pattern to be real. The pediatrician studies the page, suggests steadying dinner, trimming triggers, and guarding sleep while they wait for referrals. In two weeks, the night terrors fall to once a week. In a month, they're rare. Mornings soften. Nothing miraculous, only rhythm restored because someone paused long enough to see the map in her hands.

These three rooms matter as much as the first one. They show what the system looks like when a clinician chooses presence over protocol, when curiosity outlasts the checklist, and when the parent's pattern gets treated as data rather than noise. The system produced all four visits on the same morning. The difference in outcome traces back to one variable: whether the person in the white coat decided to slow down. That decision is always available, and it runs on nothing more than a clinician who remembers which clock their patient is actually on.

This is the window that matters, because the developing brain is pliable. A six-month wait is six months of pruning, not simply a pause. Circuits shape around absence, around the words that vanish and the gaze that slips away. Eventually, doors close that won't open the same way again.

Neurodevelopment hinges on timing. The brain sculpts itself hour by hour, pruning connections that don't fire and reinforcing those that do. Circuits for connection form and refine early, and if they falter without a response, the brain builds around the gap instead. Synapses don't hold for paperwork. Time decides outcome.

Beneath the surface, the body's already shifting. For fragile wiring, each unrecognized week compounds the load. Cumulative stress and cellular friction wear down neural pathways. Nutrients run thin and inflammatory signals rise as the toddler's brain fights to keep pace. He looks the same, but the chemistry's already different, and none of it shows up in a quick screen.

We call these visits well checks, but most are administrative rituals: a measurement, a weight, a few scripted questions that weren't built to hold genuine surveillance. What they should be is time. Room for story rather than boxes. A place where parents can speak without interruption, and space for concern that doesn't yet fit a label. The exam should also include the parent's knowing: the catch in a sentence, the way a mother circles back to the same detail because that's where the fear lives. She doesn't often carry the vocabulary of cellular disruption, but she carries the clock. The brain sculpts itself while she waits for a callback, and she's living the biology in real time even if the chart won't name it.

The system isn't tuned to that frequency. It hears only what fits the frame: a chief complaint, a code, a pathway to reimbursement. Everything else gets filtered out. And so the first flicker of miswiring gets missed, the quiet warning passes unremarked, and the sign that the window's narrowing slips by unnamed. That's what Big Medicine makes too easy: the moment that could change everything passes quietly, because the system was never designed to catch it. The clinicians in those three morning rooms didn't have a better system. They had a better minute, and that minute was enough.

The doctor enters the exam room with three rules pressed into habit. Open with the stated complaint. Complete the measurable exam. Move the plan. Training rewards speed, but early signals don't. The parent tries to pivot from ears to words, but her sentence collides with a protocol built for nose, throat, and lungs. The exam comes back clean, and in comes the false relief. We've taught ourselves to trust what we can measure fast over what emerges over time.

She finally says it: "He stopped saying mama. He doesn't turn to his name." The room shivers. The doctor understands the gravity of regression, but the system rewards speed over pause. With a full schedule and a screen demanding attention, he settles on a familiar conclusion: there's a wide range of normal. True in a lecture hall, that range becomes false when a child is losing ground. It was built for context, not as protection against change. The plan prints as the door opens, and the moment closes with it.

The minute that mattered sat between 9:01 and 9:02. It held the story, the pattern, and the chance to act before biology hardened. That minute is easy to miss, but it's still where outcomes bend.

Presence can still win inside this frame. It sounds like this: "Tell me more."

The parent says: "He had about twenty words before, but then they started to fade. Mama went first. The pauses between his speech grew longer. Now he doesn't turn to his name, and he seems farther away."

The clinician replies: "This sounds like regression, and regression is serious."

Three moves follow, and none of them require a diagnosis. Date the loss. Protect sleep and steady fuel to safeguard pruning. Then order the next actionable steps immediately: developmental assessment now, early-intervention referral today, hearing screen this week. If spells or stares live in the story, start the path to an EEG. If sleep hints at iron deficiency, check ferritin. If the parent's map ties food to sleepless nights, act on it while you wait. This is how you keep plasticity plastic.

A resident once told me the thing he feared most in clinic wasn't the seizure or the fever. It was the parent's whisper at minute twelve. He'd feel the checklist pull him forward while the parent pulled him back. He wasn't unkind. He was outnumbered: by the schedule, the screen, and the culture. He wanted a sentence that let him widen the visit without apology, so I gave him one to carry: "Let's slow down and start at the beginning." He used it twice the next day. Both times the visit slowed, both times the plan changed, and both times the parent cried from relief that someone had finally stopped to listen.

The things that shift the course are simple: a moment, a pattern, and a witness. A moment makes time visible. A pattern shows where the story's headed. A witness gives shape to memory. Parents carry the record, and clinicians can ask for it: "Help me see what happens at home. Walk me through yesterday from dawn to bedtime." What medicine calls soft is often the only thing hard enough to change wiring before the window closes.

When the room is rushing, a parent can still anchor the minute with one breath. Start with when it began and what's shifted, then ask for action tied to timing: "Change started mid-August. He lost the word mama, and he doesn't turn to his name. His sleep is lighter, and meltdowns spike after late dinners. I need the next step that protects his brain while we evaluate." That's how clarity sounds.

The system bills for vaccines and vision tests, not for the minutes that save circuits or the pause that lets a story land. The risk it ignores is the one the brain pays: delay, priced into the day, spread across the schedule, and charged to the child.

There's a reason parents leave rooms with a lump of unsaid words in their throat. They felt the minute pass, the window shift, and the plan step over what mattered because the plan had somewhere else to be. We built a culture that praises clean notes more than clear stories. We built a pace that closes visits faster than it opens windows. We let the clock decide instead of the child, and we call it caution.

Asking a toddler's brain to idle is a decision to let pruning take what it can't give back. In pediatrics, time is a clinical variable, and waiting on change carries its own cost. The visit is brief. The stakes aren't.

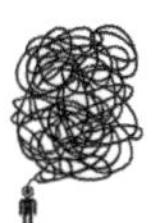

CHAPTER 24

THE CODE AND THE CLOCK

THE DOOR CLOSES, but the story doesn't stop. What happens next unfolds behind closed doors, in back offices and boardrooms parents never see.

The pediatrician clicks through the chart, enters a code, and the parent's alarm becomes the language of reimbursement. The child is no longer a toddler whose words have vanished. He's a billing line, a routine visit with a notation about possible delay. That code decides what comes next: what tests can be ordered, which referrals approved, how fast the process moves. Behind those keystrokes sits the machinery that decides how long a parent must wait while a child's brain miswires itself in real time. Every rule that governs the process was written to manage cost, not protect plasticity.

Parents imagine insurance as a safety net. In reality, it's the architect of access and the gatekeeper of time. It decides whether a symptom deserves urgency or should idle until signs turn dramatic. Cumulative stress doesn't pause because a claim is pending. Sleep loss doesn't soften because prior authorization is slow. Genes and wiring vulnerabilities keep setting thresholds while the clock runs, and for children born with immune quirks or inherited susceptibilities, every week of delay carries a higher biological price.

Insurers are built to minimize expense. "Medical necessity" means justifiable by preset criteria written to avoid cost, not criteria written to protect a child's brain. The same algorithm that approves a middle-aged man's knee MRI decides whether a toddler's lost language deserves an EEG. The same rubric that governs adult dermatology referrals gets applied to a child's regression. The gap between what biology demands and what insurers permit is where miswiring takes root.

A fifteen-month-old girl stops clapping. Three months later, she stops singing. Her mother brings her in, uneasy. That mother was me. The pediatrician notices a shift and requests a developmental evaluation. Insurance denies it as not medically necessary and directs the family to try developmental therapy first, then occupational therapy. While the family complies, neurons keep disconnecting and inflammatory signals rise. Her genes have already set a thin cellular reserve, and delay seals it completely. By the time she reaches developmental pediatrics, the visit ends in a label: autism. The miswiring continues. Neurology enters the frame only when seizures become undeniable, and about a year later, genetic testing finally names the truth. Biology keeps moving while the system stalls.

I didn't misread it. I just couldn't outrun it.

Insurers want proof before action: codes rather than intuition, objective data rather than the knot in a parent's stomach. But by the time data are objective enough for an algorithm, cellular strain has been corroding wiring for months. For fragile brains, that time is irretrievable. Waiting for certainty compounds damage.

When the system calls caution what parents live as loss, parents fight back. They learn which codes unlock approval. They sit on hold. They appeal denials and submit letters and research articles, translating fear into documentation. Some win. Most don't. The machinery is designed to wear them down. Each denial saves money, each delay shifts the burden of proof, and while parents fight, biology keeps moving. Every pending claim writes itself into a child's wiring. Every delay becomes anatomy.

When a family is told to return in six months, they're being asked to accept six months of pruning, six months of cumulative disruption, and six months of fragile wiring bending under stress. They're being asked to trade biology for bureaucracy. Time lost to paperwork is time the brain can't replace.

Parents sense this. They feel the tick of a clock no one else acknowledges, and they push because they intuitively know what delay costs. Every day without action deepens the rut. Every week without intervention makes the circuit harder to reclaim. Yet the system pathologizes that urgency. Call a third time, and you're persistent. Push for a referral, and you're anxious. Appeal a denial, and you're difficult. In the chart, your advocacy becomes character: worried, demanding, noncompliant. Rarely is it recorded for what it actually is, the most accurate diagnostic signal available.

That's how Big Medicine writes itself into a child's story: through erosion of trust. It makes the parent feel like the obstacle and makes the mother doubt what her body knows. While doubt spreads, neural strain compounds and circuits falter. The chart grows, but understanding doesn't.

Biology is relentless. It doesn't respect prior authorization, pause for insurance review, or stop while you fight through hold music. Yet the system behaves as if time is infinite, as if the developing brain can wait. If we were serious about protecting children's wiring, we'd treat parental concern as urgent data. We'd shorten the path to evaluation rather than stretching it into months. We'd act on suspicion rather than demanding certainty, because in neurodevelopment, certainty often arrives too late.

Imagine a different system. A parent reports skill loss in a child under five. The clinician marks a fast-track code: regression observed. Within forty-eight hours, early-intervention contact is made. Insurance covers interim supports: sleep stabilization, nutrition consult, developmental screening. Neurology triage runs in parallel rather than in sequence. Documentation continues, but action starts immediately. The cost of early response would be far lower than the lifelong expense of untreated miswiring. But the machinery runs on delayed validation rather than prevention, so the window keeps closing while the system verifies the obvious.

Parents already serve as the bridge the system refuses to build. They share notes between specialists, fax lab results twice, and remind providers who's waiting on whom. They build continuity by force of will. The medical record system calls this redundancy. It's survival. Every hour they spend coordinating is another hour the brain sculpts itself, indifferent to the inbox queue.

I once watched a mother in clinic read an insurance denial aloud while holding her toddler on her lap. The letter said there wasn't enough documentation of loss to justify additional evaluation. The child sat silent, eyes vacant, tracing the doctor's stethoscope cord. The mother said, "He can't wait six more weeks." She wasn't wrong. Every day he lived inside that denial, circuits kept pruning. The pediatrician glanced at the schedule, twenty minutes until the next patient, then opened the chart to annotate the loss the insurer claimed wasn't documented. By the time approval arrived, the child had lost six more words.

The cruelty isn't always visible. It hides in form letters and policy language, in words like pending, routine, and authorization required. Parents learn the dialect of delay: that routine can mean six months, that pending can mean we don't want to pay. And they translate these euphemisms into biology: years of struggle, and a window of brain plasticity quietly closing.

The paradox is brutal. The system meant to protect children's health converts biology into paperwork, and the more fragile the wiring, the less compatible the child becomes with the tempo of cost containment. What's urgent for the brain remains optional for the ledger. Delay reshapes families. Parents learn to document and advocate, becoming case managers before their children start kindergarten. What the system calls empowerment is survival dressed as compliance.

If we understood timing as biology, we'd rewrite every rule. We'd recognize that acting on early patterns saves more than waiting for proof. We'd measure the cost of delay in neurons rather than dollars, and we'd design the machinery to match the tempo of development rather than the tempo of billing. We haven't done that yet.

So the cycle continues: parents keep waiting while their children lose the one resource biology never returns. Time.

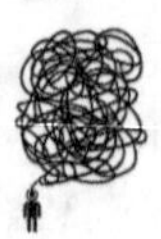

CHAPTER 25

THE PARENT AS BIOMARKER

YOU FEEL it the moment you sit down. The tilt of the head, the polite half-smile, fingers already poised over the keyboard before you finish your first sentence. Every word you speak is weighed for tone as much as content. Speak too softly, and you're dismissed. Speak too firmly, and you're labeled. Cry, and you're too emotional. Ask too many questions, and you're fixated. The balance is delicate: calm enough to be credible, insistent enough to be heard. Every sentence becomes negotiation.

It happens because medical training still runs on old assumptions: objectivity is pure, and emotion contaminates. Students are taught to trust numbers over narratives and data points over story arcs. Parental concern is treated as noise rather than data because it comes wrapped in feeling. But biology unfolds in time and context, and detachment may make for clean notes while leading to missed opportunity when the signals are subtle and the wiring still pliable.

I've watched this pattern repeat. A mother brings her toddler to the ER for blank stares that look like daydreams. The child is fine on paper: vitals normal, labs clean. The team reassures, but she presses because something isn't right. By morning, her child's chart carries a new line: Mom very anxious. That label sticks for months, and every clinician who opens the record sees it before they see her concern. Eventually, testing shows frequent absence seizures, small interruptions carving deep grooves into brain circuits. This mother's anxiety was data, not distortion.

In a child's earliest years, a parent's narrative is often the most sensitive measure available. It samples thousands of moments: sleep, food, stress, and play. It sees the whole pattern rather than the fifteen-minute slice. Inside the system, it's discounted because it isn't easily measurable, and the result is predictable: by the time evidence becomes undeniable, the child's biology has already shifted its course. This is the cost of treating parental concern as contamination.

Bias deepens the gap. If you're Black, your concern is less likely to be believed. If English isn't your first language, your accuracy is halved by translation and your urgency sanded down between sentences. If you're young, new to parenting, or alone, credibility falls before you speak. I've seen parents sit beside interpreters, speaking in short bursts while another voice carries their fear across the room. The words arrive, but the urgency thins. Details get edited out because they sound odd or superstitious. "He screams after bread and then goes quiet for hours." The meaning disappears between languages.

The paperwork structure amplifies the gap: chief complaint, brief history, exam, plan. Your story must compress to fit the form, and by the time it's typed, it's been rerouted through categories that flatten what you lived. A meltdown becomes misbehavior. Gagging at dinner becomes picky eating. Toe-walking becomes a quirk. The map you carry never makes it into the record.

I've sat with hundreds of parents after these visits, and the same ache repeats across accents and rooms. They describe moments that felt small until they weren't: a gaze that slipped, a laugh that turned brittle, a child who stopped climbing or calling for them. They were measuring time in a way the system doesn't. Children don't live in charts. They live in bodies that change fast. A three-month delay in a toddler is a neurological season, a cycle of connection and refinement that closes whether or not anyone is watching. Doctors often miss these signals because they've been trained to filter them out. Medicine didn't start detached. It was taught to be.

The roots go back a century. In 1847, the newly formed American Medical Association centralized power to raise standards and curb fraud, but centralization shifted allegiance upward, and the exam room began answering to hierarchy more than humanity. In 1910, the Carnegie Foundation funded the Flexner Report, a document that reshaped medical education under Rockefeller and Carnegie influence. Schools teaching community medicine, midwifery, and holistic care were shut down. Black medical colleges were erased. Women healers and midwives were driven out. What was measurable survived, and what was relational disappeared. In 1965, Medicare and Medicaid expanded access and millions gained entry, but fee-for-service reimbursement rewarded volume over presence. The doctor's time became the system's liability, and the fifteen-minute visit was born. In 1997, direct-to-consumer pharmaceutical advertising was legalized, pills became brands overnight, and doctors were squeezed between insurers demanding speed and parents arriving pre-scripted by commercials. Time shrank again as attention split, and the body's subtler languages fell silent.

By then, medicine had lost the ability to see the child whole. Each reform tightened the frame until a child's lived story no longer fit. None of these reforms aimed to harm. The system simply forgot what couldn't be coded. Still, the biology never changed.

Bring the lens back and biology clarifies. Loss of words after viral illness points to inflammation and metabolic pressure destabilizing fragile synapses. Night terrors clustered after late dinners point to fuel volatility and stress chemistry spilling into sleep. Meltdowns following crowded rooms point to sensory overload and autonomic strain. Eczema flaring with dairy and heat points to histamine burden and skin-barrier load. None of this requires a diagnosis to begin stabilizing. Intentional steps can reduce cellular injury while deeper evaluation proceeds.

That's why the parent's voice should be treated as a biomarker. It carries longitudinal data, and a parent carries the long arc, positioned to notice early deviation before it registers on a chart. The system is meant to amplify that signal and move a plan forward. Until cooperation becomes the baseline posture, it helps to lead with essentials when you enter the room. Change began on this date. Lost skills, listed plainly. Systems involved: skin, gut, sleep, behavior. Frequency at home. Family history, stated directly. And then: I'm asking for evaluation now because timing affects wiring. Then stop, and let silence work for you.

That shift saves time and neural capacity. It saves parents years of wondering whether they pushed hard enough, and it protects children from the irreversible cost of waiting for certainty. Put the parent back in the center, and biology responds. It always has.

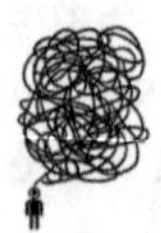

CHAPTER 26

THE BODY DOESN'T SPEAK IN SILOS

WHAT HISTORY BUILT, billing still rewards.

She came for the rash. It began on his cheeks, red and dry, and crept behind his knees. The pediatrician glanced, prescribed a cream, and moved on, with a handout on gentle cleansers and a note about possible allergens. Just eczema. Three weeks later, she came back for constipation: straining, hard stools, four or five days between bowel movements. Probably diet, the pediatrician said. More water, more fiber, maybe a stool softener. A referral was considered, then deferred. Two months after that, she returned because everything felt louder. Her child clung in crowded rooms, resisted transitions, and sleep fractured into shards. Probably just a phase, she was told. Kids get clingy. Give it time.

Each visit read like a separate story, each symptom handled in isolation: skin, gut, then brain. Different boxes, different codes, and never a single thread pulled through. But she sensed a bigger picture, her child's body sounding the alarm in multiple languages at once. She didn't have a medical degree, but she felt the pattern, and she knew something was going unseen.

Medicine calls it systems-based care. It looks efficient and organized, and for children it can be devastating. It survives because it fits the billing logic: separate problems are easier to code than connected ones. Efficiency wins reimbursement, and connection doesn't. But the body doesn't speak in silos, least of all a child's. Distress rarely stays in one lane. When the gut is inflamed, the skin often flares. When sleep falters, regulation often spirals. When fuel wobbles, attention often cracks. The metabolic, immune, and nervous systems talk constantly, and modern medicine cuts that conversation into parts.

That's how early miswiring hides in plain sight. Stress chemistry and metabolic strain creep in, rhythms break, and miswiring flickers across systems: eczema here, constipation there, meltdowns everywhere. None of those signals alone rings loud, but together they describe a body under pressure. For a child carrying genetic variants that touch synapses, mitochondria, or immune signaling, that strain rises faster and recedes slower.

Fragmented care becomes a risk factor in its own right. Fragmentation brings polydoctoring: dermatology for the skin, gastroenterology for the gut, psychiatry for the mind. Each specialist owns a slice and no one claims the whole. One calls it inflammatory, another metabolic, another behavioral. Each is partly right, and none is complete. While the system stalls, time does its work. Disrupted rhythms deepen, neurons adapt around absence, and circuits lay detours that are harder to unbuild. What could have been caught early gets scattered, and the body writes its story toward permanence.

This is why so many parents feel that things don't add up, and why children get labeled complex when the complexity belongs to the framework. I've seen parents try to connect the dots themselves when no one else would. One mother taped index cards across a wall, sleep on one, spells on another, and connected them wherever patterns overlapped. A father tracked his son's tantrums and saw they rose in lockstep with the days his gut slowed. Another mother kept photos of skin flare-ups beside notes on heat and sugar. None had medical training, but all saw patterns the system missed. It's rarely the parent who's fragmented.

The tragedy is that their insight doesn't register until the child is significantly off course. By the time professionals integrate the pieces, the brain may have closed doors that won't open the same way again. The answer isn't more specialists or more codes. It's coherence. What do skin, gut, and mood share? How do sleep, food, and stress chemistry press on the same circuits? Eczema, constipation, and anxiety aren't usually three unrelated problems in the same body. They're more often byproducts of one storm: cumulative stress and metabolic friction corroding wiring, triggered by genetic sensitivity and intensified by broken rhythm. This is physiology, not complexity. When parents voice patterns across systems, they're offering the synthesis that specialties rarely claim.

Unrelieved strain shifts a child's internal rhythm long before it produces findings that any single specialty can name. Fragmentation turns shared physiology into separate problems, and the pattern disappears in the handoffs. To protect our children's wiring, we have to keep their body whole. Systems are puzzle pieces. Kids aren't.

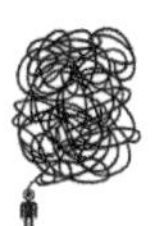

CHAPTER 27

YOU WEREN'T IMAGINING IT

YOU LIVED THE EARLY SHIFT. Hour by hour, meal by meal, bedtime after bedtime, you were reading your child's biology as it unfolded in real time, through the texture of ordinary days that the system would later reduce to checkboxes and percentiles. The change you felt was real. The unease you carried into waiting rooms was accurate. The pattern you traced across weeks of mornings and evenings and sleepless midnights was data, and it was yours long before anyone with credentials agreed to look at it.

Whether you're a mother, a father, a grandparent, a foster parent, an aunt, an uncle, a sibling, or a cousin, your body flags the shift before language does. A sudden silence where there was sound. A gaze that used to find yours and now slides past. Tantrums that escalate past what the day seems to warrant and then collapse into something that looks less like anger than exhaustion. These are signatures of cellular dysfunction, and the moment you registered them, even the moment you registered them as a feeling you couldn't yet name, was a moment of genuine diagnostic perception. The fact that it arrived through your body rather than through a chart doesn't make it less precise. It makes it earlier.

What rarely makes it into the record is who you actually are in relation to your child: someone who has been paying sustained, daily attention across months and years, tracking the arc of a developing nervous system through proximity that no clinician's appointment can replicate. You've watched this child wake and eat and play and fall apart and recover across thousands of ordinary moments. You carry that dataset in your body. In the earliest years of a child's life, that embodied longitudinal record is one of the most sensitive diagnostic instruments available, and the system discounts it almost by reflex, treating story as noise and pattern as anxiety and the parent's knowing as something to be managed rather than something to be heard.

The mechanism behind that discounting is structural rather than personal. Medical training still runs largely on the assumption that objectivity lives in numbers and subjectivity contaminates them, which means parental concern arrives in the exam room pre-labeled as distortion. A mother who pushes past reassurance is anxious. A father who comes in with documentation is difficult. A grandparent who insists something has changed is projecting. The label attaches before the content is examined, and once it's in the chart, every clinician who opens the record sees the label before they see the concern. The concern gets filtered through the label rather than considered on its own terms, and the child's biology keeps moving while the adults in the room debate the parent's credibility.

That's a costly debate. Your child's developmental arc doesn't pause for it. The brain sculpts itself through the weeks it takes to get a referral approved and the months it takes for an appointment to arrive, pruning connections that aren't firing and reinforcing the ones that are, indifferent to what's pending in the system. For a child whose wiring is already fragile, those weeks and months carry a biological price that compounds in ways no single later intervention can fully recover. Timing is a clinical variable in neurodevelopment, and the system behaves as though it's administrative. The distance between those two understandings of time is where miswiring takes root and deepens while paperwork churns.

Parents are told that if they would simply trust the process, the process would deliver what their child needs. The process was built to manage cost and volume, and those are genuinely difficult problems. But a developing brain is neither a cost center nor a volume unit, and the parent standing at the intersection of their child's biology and the system's throughput model is doing something the system wasn't designed to accommodate: holding complexity that the fifteen-minute visit was built to compress away. Your voice in that room is carrying more information than the form can hold. Your pattern recognition is operating on a longer timeline than the appointment allows. Your urgency is calibrated to your child's biological clock rather than to the referral queue, and that calibration is correct.

The system will keep doing what it was built to do. Referrals will take time. Screenings will skim surfaces. Labels will arrive after windows have already narrowed. None of that changes what you saw, or when you saw it, or what it meant. You were reading something real with the most accurate instrument available: sustained, loving, daily attention to a specific nervous system you know better than anyone else on earth. The instinct you carried into that waiting room, the one that sat in your chest like a weight before you could name it, was the earliest signal in the room. It was also the most accurate one. Trust it accordingly, and let that trust be the thing that keeps you moving when the system asks you to wait.

Do This Before Your Next Appointment

Bring one page. Write your child's symptoms, sleep pattern, and food log. Hand it over at the start.

Set your priority. Decide on one question you won't leave without asking. Write it down.

Use this script. "What's the single next step that will give us the clearest insight into what's going on?"

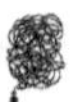

THE EXAM ROOM is downstream of decisions made far from any patient. Which tests get ordered, which referrals get approved, which concerns get logged as anxiety and which get logged as data: all of it traces back to an institution meant to safeguard children's health, now increasingly steered by the very industries it was built to restrain.

That institution is government, and its policies are already shaping the environment children are miswiring inside: the food that's federally approved, the chemicals that are legally permitted, the programs that promise protection and deliver something narrower. Part Five names what those policies actually do, and to whom.

REFERENCES

1. American Medical Association. (2025). *AMA History*. Retrieved from https://www.ama-assn.org/about/ama-history/ama-history.

2. Angell, M. (2004). *The Truth About the Drug Companies: How They Deceive Us and What to Do About It*. Random House. ISBN: 978-0375508462.

3. Brandt, S. (2022). *Women Healers: Gender, Authority, and Medicine in Early Philadelphia*. University of Pennsylvania Press. ISBN: 978-0812253863.

4. Brennan, T. A. (2024). *The Transformation of American Health Insurance: On the Path to Universal Coverage*. Johns Hopkins University Press. ISBN: 978-1421449098.

5. Brownlee, S. (2008). *Overtreated: Why Too Much Medicine Is Making Us Sicker and Poorer*. Bloomsbury. ISBN: 978-1582345796.

6. Burchett, M. (2023). Nixon Signs HMOs into Law. *EBSCO Research Starters*. Retrieved from https://www.ebsco.com/research-starters/history/nixon-signs-hmos-law.

7. Coombs, J. G. (2005). *The Rise and Fall of HMOs: An American Health Care Revolution*. University of Wisconsin Press. ISBN: 978-0299202408.

8. Crowley, J., et al. (2019). Nutrition Education in Medical Schools: A Systematic Review. *Lancet Planet Health*, 3(9):e379-e389. Retrieved from https://www.thelancet.com/journals/lanplh/article/PIIS2542-5196(19)30171-8/fulltext.

9. Dean, W. (2023). *If I Betray These Words: Moral Injury in Medicine and Why It's So Hard for Clinicians to Put Patients First*. Steerforth Press. ISBN: 978-1586423544.

10. EBSCO. (2022). First Medical School in the United States. Retrieved from https://www.ebsco.com/research-starters/education/first-medical-school-united-states.

11. Flexner, A. (1910). *Medical Education in the United States and Canada*. Carnegie Foundation. Retrieved from http://archive.carnegiefoundation.org/publications/pdfs/elibrary/Carnegie_Flexner_Report.pdf.

12. Gray, B. H. (1991). *The Profit Motive and Patient Care: The Changing Accountability of Doctors and Hospitals*. Harvard University Press.

13. Ludmerer, K. M. (2014). *Let Me Heal: The Opportunity to Preserve Excellence in American Medicine*. Oxford University Press. ISBN: 978-0199744541.

14. Makary, M. (2019). *The Price We Pay: What Broke American Health Care —and How to Fix It*. Bloomsbury Publishing. ISBN: 978-1635574111.

15. Morsy, L. (2022). Carnegie and Rockefeller's Philanthropic Legacy: Exclusion of African Americans From Medicine. Retrieved from https://pubmed.ncbi.nlm.nih.gov/36512812/.

16. Murray, J. E. (2007). *Origins of American Health Insurance: A History of Industrial Sickness Funds*. Yale University Press. ISBN: 978-0300120912.

17. Relman, A. (1980). The New Medical-Industrial Complex. *New England Journal of Medicine*, 303(17), 963–970. Retrieved from https://doi.org/10.1056/NEJM198010233031703.

18. Rosenthal, E. (2017). *An American Sickness: How Healthcare Became Big Business and How You Can Take It Back*. Penguin Press. ISBN: 978-1594206757.

19. Starr, P. (1983). *The Social Transformation of American Medicine: The Rise of a Sovereign Profession and the Making of a Vast Industry*. Basic Books. ISBN: 978-0465079346.

PART 5
BIG GOVERNMENT
A SYSTEM, NOT A GUIDELINE

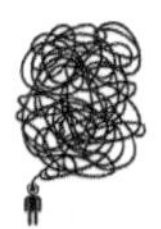

CHAPTER 28

THE TRAY THAT TEACHES THE BRAIN

IT STARTS WITH A TRAY. Beige plastic, five compartments. A rectangle of pizza that barely qualifies as bread, a scoop of canned corn, a plastic cup of chocolate milk offered like a nutrient, and maybe a bag of baked chips stamped "smart snack." The air smells of reheated starch, and the industrial warmer hums like white noise. This is lunch for tens of millions of children, by design.

That tray is the endpoint of a policy machine carrying the full weight of the federal government. We want to believe our kids are fed well, that whatever shape the food pyramid wears now springs from evidence rather than strategy, that "whole grain" means nourishment at the cellular level, that milk always builds bone, and that vegetable means fresh, green, alive. The truth is harder to swallow: the system that feeds children was built to stabilize markets and move product. What lands on the tray reflects what industry needs to sell, and children's brains pay the price.

Start with the USDA. One agency holds two mandates that should never share a roof: promote American agriculture and safeguard the nation's nutrition. That's a structural flaw with consequences. The same institution that props up corn, soy, and dairy through subsidies also writes the dietary rules that shape school menus and public feeding programs. Those menus lean on the cheapest, most abundant commodities, and a slice of refined flour topped with processed cheese and a smear of tomato paste can clear the vegetable checkbox because the regulations permit that smear to count. Cafeteria managers start with procurement lists, bid awards, and compliance targets, not a child's biology. The National School Lunch Program sets the categories, vendors pitch the cheapest ways to fill them, and districts choose items that survive transport, store well, and keep costs low. Paperwork verifies calories and components. No one measures cellular impact.

The tray clears compliance even as it loads developing brains with oxidative stress, inflammatory additives, and fuel swings that hit like a tide. Compliance is the system congratulating itself while a child's biology takes the hit.

One mother decided to see what compliance actually meant. She asked for the district's wellness policy and learned that vending machines stocked with soda and chips were considered within policy. What mattered to her wasn't whether her child bought from them. It was what the system defined as acceptable fuel for a developing brain. Seeing that standard told her everything she needed to know. She stopped trying to argue with it and protected what she could, packing lunches with fruit, protein, and water, and over time she watched her son steady.

Another parent told me her daughter fell apart after starting kindergarten. At home, she'd thrived on simple food. Weeks into school lunches, mood and sleep unraveled: daily meltdowns, loss of interest in play, night waking. The teacher called it adjustment, the pediatrician called it a phase. Meanwhile, the parent traced it back to the tray, pizza, fries, and juice, four days a week, every week. She was watching her daughter's biology react to those inputs in real time, with policy carrying out the wrong mandate perfectly.

Here's the mechanism the paperwork ignores. Cellular

disruption arises when daily inputs create more oxidative and inflammatory stress than a child can neutralize. When repair falls behind, mitochondria tire, neurons misfire, and membranes inflame as signaling frays. Fuel instability tightens the screw. The brain needs steady delivery, and flavored milk spikes insulin, refined flour becomes sugar in minutes, and snack bars laced with syrups collapse energy before the next class begins. A child who can't hold focus after lunch is simply riding the curve that policy designed.

School lunches aren't crafted by clinicians who study synaptic pruning or sleep architecture. They're engineered by policy analysts, commodity contracts, and cost calculators. Behind every entrée sits a chain of lobbying, subsidies, and procurement rules that prize shelf stability over nutrient density. The meal is built to hit caloric minimums, tick compliance boxes, and satisfy vendors. If it also floods fragile circuits with noise, no one calls that failure.

At home, the same incentives follow families into grocery aisles, and for low-income families they arrive with far less room to maneuver. SNAP, the federal food assistance program, steers purchasing toward boxed and bagged foods because those are the options the program makes most accessible and most afford-able. Fresh produce, quality protein, and healthy fats exist tech-nically within the program's rules, but they're priced out of reach for families spending every benefit dollar on volume. The system optimizes for calories, and calories are what it delivers. WIC, the federal nutrition program for women, infants, and young chil-dren, defaults to milk and cereal as its foundational offerings, whether or not a child's biology tolerates either. A toddler with immune sensitivity, gut inflammation, or a genetic variant that disrupts dairy metabolism receives the same default package as every other child in the program, because WIC wasn't designed around individual biology. It was designed around agricultural surplus and political negotiation.

The consequence falls hardest on the children who can least

afford it. Families with resources can supplement, substitute, and opt out. They can pack the lunch, choose the store, and absorb the cost of a different default. Families without those resources live inside the program's assumptions. Their children eat what the policy provides, and when those inputs destabilize developing brains, the disruption gets attributed to the child rather than the system. A low-income child who can't focus, regulate, or sleep is labeled difficult before anyone asks what they ate for breakfast. The biology is identical across income levels. The inputs aren't, and neither are the consequences. Big Government, through SNAP and WIC, doesn't just fail to protect fragile wiring. It actively funds the inputs that corrode it, at scale, among the children most biologically vulnerable to the damage.

A father came to see me exhausted. His eight-year-old melted down each afternoon around two and fought sleep every night, and school lunch meant chocolate milk, nuggets, and fries. We changed three things for one week: water instead of chocolate milk, real protein and fruit in a packed lunch, and lights out thirty minutes earlier. On day four, the teacher wrote, "Whatever you did, please keep doing it." By month's end, the meltdowns had stopped and bedtime had settled. Same child, different inputs. The brain noticed.

Food is an input, and inputs steer biology. Policy turns those inputs into defaults, defaults become culture, and culture calcifies into belief: if it's federally approved, it must be safe. In policy, though, safe rarely means safe for the developing brain. It usually means available, marketable, and cheap, and the labels carry a halo that cells don't recognize. Families who seek change learn to read the rules for what they are. They study what's written, what's required, and what's permitted. They see where a vending machine slips through a loophole, where a vegetable becomes a spoonful of processed tomato, where a milk requirement pours sugar into a child who sleeps poorly and can't focus. Then they act.

No one at the USDA or the district office is tasked with

tracking cellular disruption, and no one measures stability as an outcome of federal feeding programs. The metrics are bureaucratic: pounds moved, calories served, dollars spent. Meanwhile, the biology beneath those metrics erodes in real time. So the first move is clarity. See the tray for what it is: a policy artifact, a lesson written in processed starch, sweetened dairy, and shelf-stable convenience. Then decide what gets removed and what gets replaced. Choose the inputs your child's biology can hold. Watch what shifts. Keep what steadies.

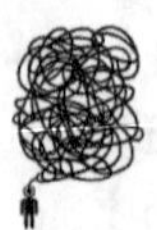

CHAPTER 29

THE BLUEPRINT BEHIND THE MENU

THE MEETING ROOM held folding chairs, a carafe of coffee, and a stack of vendor brochures. A PowerPoint listed SKUs instead of foods. The agenda read like logistics: delivery windows, storage, warm time, and portion cost. Slides flicked past while the buyer asked about case counts and crediting points. No one mentioned children.

The cafeteria isn't a kitchen. It's the distribution arm of a blueprint, and understanding that blueprint requires following the money upstream.

Federal dollars move first as entitlements. Those entitlements become USDA Foods allocated to states and then to districts. Districts issue bids, and vendors answer with SKUs engineered to meet the rules at the lowest possible cost. The menu that reaches your child is the residue of that process, a policy output rather than a nutritional intention. Products carry labels that tell a district how an item counts on the form, and crediting is what decides the winners. A slice can credit as two grain servings even if the grain is refined. A sauce can credit as a vegetable because tomato paste meets the letter of the category. Protein can arrive as a breaded patty with fillers because the label credits enough grams to fill the box. What matters to the system is that the tray adds up on paper.

Vendors engineer for this. They shape recipes to survive transport, endure storage, reheat evenly, and satisfy crediting math with the cheapest inputs available under commodity contracts. The result is food that behaves for policy and misbehaves in a child's body: steady on a pallet and erratic in a neuron.

The blueprint extends beyond the cafeteria line. Vending machines, school stores, snack lines, and à la carte options all fall under looser rules, and the products filling those spaces still push sugar, refined starch, and additives that drive sharp energy swings. Fundraisers bring in candy that clears hurdles shaped by industry negotiation rather than biology. The blueprint doesn't need to break a rule to overwhelm a child. It only has to follow what's written.

Operational gravity locks the pattern in place. Cafeteria staff are too few, training time too limited, and the equipment itself is built for reheating rather than cooking. Central kitchens push hot packs and cold packs to satellite locations with tight holding windows, so shelf-stable and frozen items win because they don't spoil the ledger. Boxes and bags beat produce that bruises and proteins that need a knife. The system favors foods that keep costs low and service on time, and the biology at the end of that chain isn't part of the calculation.

The tray looks normal because the culture insists it is, but the papers behind it tell a different story. Bid specifications limit salt and calories while permitting additives that scramble signaling. Product sheets promise whole grain after the kernel has been ground to dust. Milk rules open the door to sweetened cartons because a checkbox favors volume over stability. None of this requires malice. It requires only a system that rewards the wrong endpoints.

The blueprint lives in documents most parents never see. The wellness policy sets the local tone. The bid documents define ingredients and delivery terms. The Child Nutrition labels turn food into crediting math. The ordering lists show what's actually purchased week to week. When those documents align, the tray isn't accidental, and a child's biology absorbs the cost.

That cost compounds quietly and unevenly. A child eating five school lunches a week for the duration of an academic year absorbs more than eight hundred exposures to the inputs that policy designed. For a child with typical resilience, the cumulative load may stay subclinical, surfacing as irritability, afternoon crashes, or disrupted sleep without ever attracting a diagnosis. For a child whose wiring is already fragile, those same eight hundred exposures can tip a system already operating near its threshold. Genetic variants that affect mitochondrial efficiency, immune regulation, or neurotransmitter metabolism don't announce themselves on a cafeteria form. The tray arrives the same for every child regardless, and the gap between what a resilient nervous system can absorb and what a fragile one can't is precisely where miswiring takes root. Policy doesn't create that gap. It widens it, meal by meal, across every school day of every year.

This isn't about one slice or one carton. It's about a regulatory design that steers menus toward what stores well and prices cheaply, and away from what sustains a developing brain. The families who see it clearly are the ones who stopped waiting for the system to correct itself and started reading the documents instead. They asked for the wellness policy, pulled the bid specs, and learned the crediting rules. They saw where the loopholes lived and closed them at home as best they could.

Notice the design. Watch the cascade. And see the system choose itself.

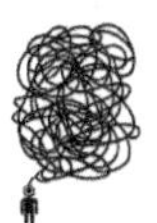

CHAPTER 30

CELLULAR DISRUPTION IN PLAIN SIGHT

PAPER RUSTLES, chairs scrape, and pencils tap. Twenty minutes after lunch, the air has shifted. One child hums to stay awake. Another folds her worksheet, eyes glazed. A boy fidgets hard enough to shake the desk. The teacher moves between them, trying to steady a rhythm that won't hold. She's witnessing biochemistry, but what she doesn't see is the policy that scripted this hour: the menu set months earlier, the bidding shaped by federal rules, and the caloric minimums that put chocolate milk and starch on every tray. The behavior looks like a classroom problem. More often, it's a fuel problem, a timing problem, and a stability problem.

Government meal programs guarantee calories, but they don't guarantee stability. Calories are easy to measure. Stability, that space between load and repair, isn't. When that margin thins, the child slips.

Post-lunch crashes follow a pattern. A child steady at ten tips into fog by one. Some go quiet while others go frantic, and a few fall apart with no warning at all. Their bodies are sending distress signals long before anyone names them. Teachers often assume the child is having a day. Clinicians assume the pattern is disorder. Parents start doubting their intuition because no one else sees what they know. But the timing is the tell.

A kindergarten teacher once told me her class unraveled around the same time every day. "It's like the room tilts," she said. She adjusted transitions, shortened lessons, and built in sensory breaks. Nothing held, because the problem lived in the fuel. The menu didn't change, so the pattern didn't change.

A parent told me her son felt like two different children, one before lunch and one after. His mornings were steady, but by one o'clock he vibrated with restlessness, by two he looked vacant, and by three he unraveled completely. The school wondered about a disorder, and the pediatrician floated medication. She packed a lunch with real food for a week, and the volatility noticeably softened. Nothing else changed.

That's the part policy never accounted for: the way certain inputs amplify a child's existing vulnerabilities. A child with ADHD still has ADHD. A child with oppositional tendencies still has a complex behavioral profile. But a child with fragile wiring given a menu engineered around shelf stability and caloric minimums will struggle more, because the inputs make the day harder to hold. Policy is built around procurement cycles, commodity prices, and calorie math. The school day runs on a different clock, and that mismatch surfaces in the early afternoon, when warning notes go home and phones start ringing. The child is read as defiant following a crash that was engineered in the cafeteria.

Fuel instability is only one layer, but it's a predictable one. Refined grains convert to glucose quickly. Sweetened milk amplifies the spike. Additives increase inflammatory stress, and highly processed fats place additional strain on cell membranes. None of these effects are catastrophic in isolation, but stacked day after day, tray after tray, they narrow the biological margin a child depends on. Some children have wide margins. Some don't.

A government-approved meal can deliver calories while

eroding stability. On paper, everything looks adequate. In practice, neurons are white-knuckling through the afternoon. Children who genuinely need support still need it, but engineered instability becomes the backdrop against which every symptom plays out. Patterns driven by fuel and timing get mistaken for disorder, and supports that should begin in the environment drift toward medication by default.

This isn't the teacher's fault, or the clinician's, or the parent's. The architecture is doing exactly what it was built to do: track inputs and outputs rather than children. It moves pallets and calories and leaves developing biology to fend for itself. No agency is charged with guarding coherence or tracking the arc of a child's day. The metrics that would signal real trouble, inflammatory load and repair capacity, never enter the forms that drive decisions. What remains are artifacts of collapse: behavior notes, phone calls home, and prescriptions that capture the fallout while leaving the cause untouched.

For some children, the cafeteria is the first place their vulnerabilities get amplified. For others, it's where their diagnosis gets misframed. For almost everyone, it becomes a steady drip of instability that no one traces back to the tray. The outcome follows the design.

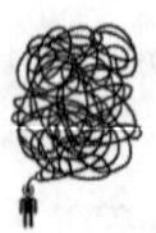

CHAPTER 31

THE ILLUSION OF SAFETY

EVERY PARENT WANTS to believe the system screens what goes into a child's body. If something were truly dangerous, it wouldn't be allowed. If it's on the shelf, it must be safe. If it's served in schools, it must have passed inspection. That belief steadies us when time is short and life is crowded. But practice says otherwise.

Federal oversight doesn't mean active protection of the developing nervous system. It offers no guarantee that early exposures won't derail long-term brain development, and it doesn't test for the conditions that drive cellular disruption. In this system, "safe" has a legal meaning rather than a biological one. It means permissible. It means tolerable risk. The question regulators ask isn't whether something harms the brain. It's how much harm is acceptable, and whose risk gets prioritized. The answer, built into the architecture of the system, is industry's.

Consider food additives: the dyes that make yogurt fluorescent pink, the emulsifiers that hold dressings together, the preservatives that stretch shelf life. Some were never meaningfully tested for safety in humans, adults or children alike. Under a regulatory clause called "Generally Recognized as Safe," companies can self-certify a chemical's safety without independent review. A manufacturer convenes its own panel, cites decades-old studies, and files nothing with the FDA. Most compounds stay approved and invisible, and proactive reviews are rare. Harm usually has to surface before anyone looks.

That's how additives like butylated hydroxyanisole, butylated hydroxytoluene, and polysorbate 80 still circulate in snacks and cereals marketed to children. They passed paper safety reviews because no one asked the question that matters most: what do they do to developing neurons under daily exposure?

The same logic governs pesticides. The Environmental Protection Agency sets residue limits one chemical at a time, without accounting for how children actually eat: cereal sprayed with glyphosate, fruit dusted with fungicides, milk from cows exposed to antibiotics. Each exposure is judged in isolation, but the biology absorbing them isn't. Load accumulates, and the developing brain bears the cost. Certain organophosphate pesticides are linked to measurable IQ loss and structural changes in children's brains. Chlorpyrifos stayed legal for years after those patterns emerged, until lawsuits and headlines finally forced its withdrawal. Protection arrived after the damage, as it so often does.

A mother once told me her son's tantrums spiked after brightly colored yogurt tubes. The pediatrician called it coincidence, but she trusted what she observed. When she removed the dyes, the rages stopped. No trial, no grant, just observation and repair. Her data never entered the record.

The thresholds that define safe exposure are built around adult weight, adult metabolism, and adult resilience. They ignore the developmental windows when neurons prune and detox pathways are still immature. They don't account for genetic vulnerabilities: a weaker glutathione pathway, slower energy output, thinner membranes. And they don't account for stacking, the way dozens of small exposures combine until the cumulative load exceeds what a fragile system can clear. That's how a child can eat an approved lunch, play on an approved field, and drink approved water, and still end up destabilized. Each input cleared the threshold on its own. Together, they didn't.

What's allowed isn't safe. It's permitted. The distinction is the damage.

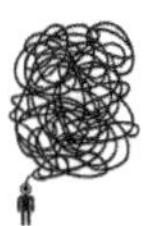

CHAPTER 32

MANAGED INEQUALITY

EQUITY LIVES on banners and press releases. It anchors mission statements and annual reports, promises fairness, protection, and shared responsibility, and on paper it looks like compassion made structural. The language is careful and the intentions, in many cases, are genuine. What the language can't do is change the architecture underneath it, and that architecture was built around a different set of priorities than the ones the banners name.

Nowhere is that clearer than in how the system treats vulnerable children.

Medicaid claims to level the healthcare field, and for millions of families it provides access that would otherwise be impossible. That's real and it matters. But access to a system is different from access to timely, coherent, biologically responsive care, and Medicaid delivers the first far more reliably than the second. The gap between those two things is where children's development actually lives. A child in a well-resourced home can see a developmental pediatrician within weeks, travel across state lines for a specialist whose waitlist is shorter, and assemble a care team that communicates with each other. A child on Medicaid can wait a year for an initial evaluation, longer for a follow-up, and longer still for therapy services that the law technically guarantees but that providers don't deliver because the reimbursement rate makes delivery economically impossible. Parents call daily, leave messages that go unreturned, and move up waiting lists that advance more slowly than their child's developmental windows close. The paperwork churns and the synapses prune, and the system records both as separate processes with no meaningful relationship to each other.

The reimbursement structure is where the gap gets engineered rather than merely permitted. Medicaid pays providers a fraction of what private insurance pays for the same service, and providers respond rationally to that reality by limiting the number of Medicaid patients they accept, by shortening appointment times, and by concentrating in geographic areas where the patient mix sustains a practice financially. The result is a two-tier system that uses the same language of care across both tiers while delivering fundamentally different things. A child whose biology is most fragile, whose genetic vulnerabilities are most pronounced, whose environment is already applying the most pressure, is the child most likely to be waiting longest for the evaluation that could name what's happening and begin addressing it. That's the managed part of managed inequality: it's a predictable outcome of structural choices, sustained by inertia rather than malice, and it lands with the precision of intention even when the intention was something else entirely.

Food tells the same story through a different mechanism. SNAP and WIC exist to prevent hunger, and they do. Children in families receiving these benefits eat more reliably than they would without them, and that matters in ways that are straightforward and important. But preventing hunger and supporting a developing nervous system are related goals that the programs treat as identical, and the distance between them is where the biological cost accumulates. Hunger is measured in calories and the programs are built around caloric adequacy, which means the metric they optimize for is the one least connected to synaptic pruning, mitochondrial function, inflammatory load, and the fuel stability that a developing brain requires to wire itself correctly. In affluent neighborhoods, families can supplement benefits with farmers' markets, with cleaner grocery options, with the time and kitchen infrastructure to prepare food from ingredients rather than from packages. In under-resourced communities, families buy what the program's purchasing power and the local food landscape make available, which is reliably weighted toward refined starches, sweetened dairy, and shelf-stable products that keep costs low and inflammatory burden high. The federal programs that promise to protect children's health actively fund inputs that corrode it, at the largest scale, among the children whose biology is least equipped to absorb the damage and most dependent on the system getting it right.

The early intervention and special education systems operate under the same structural logic. Federal law guarantees support, and in that guarantee lives a real promise: that a child whose development diverges from the typical trajectory has a legal right to services designed to address that divergence. What a child actually receives, though, depends almost entirely on geography, on the advocacy capacity of their family, and on the district's interpretation of words like appropriate and sufficient, words the law uses but does not define tightly enough to prevent wildly different readings. In wealthier districts, parents arrive at IEP meetings with independent evaluations, educational attorneys, and detailed knowledge of what the law requires. They push timelines, document denials, and secure services that approach what their child's biology actually needs. In poorer districts, evaluations arrive late, the goals written into plans are modest, therapy hours are fewer, and the staff delivering services turn over fast enough that continuity is a theoretical concept rather than a lived experience. The law defines appropriate and the budget defines enough, and the child's development proceeds inside the gap between those two definitions, adapting to what's available rather than to what would have been possible under different conditions.

The gap isn't abstract and it isn't neutral. Language circuits depend on rapid, repeated, responsive input during windows that close on their own biological schedule regardless of what's pending in an administrator's inbox. A child receiving fifty hours of quality speech therapy during a critical period arrives at kindergarten in a different place than a child who received fifteen hours of inconsistent service across the same span. The disability may be identical. The trajectory diverges, and the divergence becomes the child's reality rather than an administrative artifact, a permanent feature of their development rather than a consequence of a policy choice made in a building they've never entered.

That reality is distributed with a consistency that deserves to be called a pattern. Black and brown disabled children are disciplined more and suspended more, which means they're removed from the learning environments they're already receiving less support in, compounding an already compounded disadvantage. They're identified later for services, meaning the windows that early intervention is designed to reach are already narrower by the time help arrives. They're more likely to be placed in restrictive settings and less likely to be included in general education environments where the social and linguistic exposure supports the development the services are meant to build. The data on each of these disparities is extensive and consistent and has been for decades, and the pace of remedy has borne no relationship to the weight of the evidence. The disparity persists because it's been absorbed into the ordinary functioning of the system, treated as an ambient condition rather than an active choice, which is one of the more sophisticated ways a system can sustain harm while maintaining the appearance of neutrality.

Cumulative disadvantage is cellular before it's sociological. Every missed therapy session leaves a trace in the neural pathways that the session would have reinforced. Every low-nutrient meal shifts the inflammatory baseline that determines how much cognitive reserve a child has available for learning. Every prolonged stress response without adequate repair time rewires stress circuitry toward hypervigilance in ways that affect attention, memory, and social processing for years beyond the stressor itself. These effects aren't metaphorical. They accumulate in the same tissues, along the same molecular pathways, through the same biological mechanisms as any other form of chronic stress, and they compound across developmental time in ways that no single later intervention can fully reverse once the windows that made early change possible have closed.

Systems designed to equalize end up institutionalizing the opposite when their metrics are wrong, their funding is inequitable, and their enforcement is shaped by the same social hierarchies they were meant to correct. The banner stays up. The language of equity circulates. The gap widens underneath it, measured in neurons and windows and the quietly diverging trajectories of children whose biology was identical at the starting line.

This is what policy optimized for optics produces: the appearance of fairness and the architecture of its opposite, sustained by the distance between what the system says it does and what a child's developing brain actually receives.

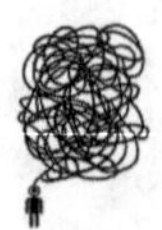

CHAPTER 33

THE FILTER ON SCIENCE

WE'RE TOLD to trust the science. The phrase lands like a command, as if science were a monument instead of a method. Real science invites challenge and correction. It doesn't live in marble, and it was never meant to live in funding cycles, institutional loyalties, or markets that decide which truths rise and which stay buried.

Consider how new drugs reach the market. Parents assume FDA approval means rigorous, independent review, but most of the data the agency sees comes from studies funded by the companies selling the drug. Trials are often short, and they measure symptom shifts rather than long-term neurodevelopment. A stimulant can improve focus on paper, but the same study rarely follows what happens to sleep architecture years later, or to resilience during critical wiring windows. The question being answered and the question that matters are often not the same question.

Nutrition science moves through the same filter. The USDA's dietary guidelines cite research funded by commodity groups with a direct stake in remaining essential. Dairy boards bankroll studies that keep milk framed as indispensable, even though many children, particularly children of color, show no meaningful bone benefit and sometimes experience inflammation. Meanwhile, research linking certain ingredients to oxidative stress or altered signaling sits at the margins, underfunded and underreported, because it doesn't pay to pursue it.

When inconvenient findings do surface, they're softened by language. Agencies write "may be associated" or "evidence is inconclusive." The phrasing is strategic, preserving public trust while deferring action. What it means in practice is that the data is strong enough to generate concern but not strong enough, in the system's accounting, to justify the cost of acting on it.

Parents live in the gap between study design and daily life. They watch a child's focus unravel after a school lunch, see calmer nights after cutting a sweetened drink, and hear laughter return once dyes leave the pantry. When they share those observations, they're told the evidence is merely anecdotal, because no trial follows a child through thousands of exposures across years of development. The absence of that trial is presented as a reason to doubt the parent. It would be more honest to treat it as a reason to run the trial.

That gap is intentional. It allows harm to persist without looking like neglect. Funding decides which questions get asked, policy decides which answers shape guidelines, and market pressure decides which findings reach the podium. Meanwhile, parents generate the longest-running dataset in existence: uncontrolled, inconvenient, and true. Their observations don't fit the form, but they're tracking what the funded studies are designed to miss.

You don't have to choose between believing science and believing yourself. Science at its best is a tool for refining observation, and your observations are data. Interrogate both, and trust the one that keeps your child steady.

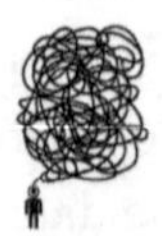

CHAPTER 34

PROTECTION THAT ARRIVES LATE

WE'VE SEEN this pattern before. Lead in paint and pipes. Bisphenol A in baby bottles. Phthalates in toys and vinyl flooring and the soft plastic surfaces of products designed specifically for children's hands and mouths. Each was declared safe. Each was defended with studies that asked narrow questions over short timeframes and found no basis for concern within the limits of what the study was designed to detect. Each was restricted only after harm became undeniable, after the epidemiology reached a threshold of consensus that the political and economic cost of continued inaction finally exceeded. Profits were secured across those years of delay. Children absorbed the biological cost of them. This sequence has repeated often enough to be recognized as pattern rather than coincidence, and patterns that repeat reliably deserve to be examined as features rather than failures.

Regulation in America is built around proof of harm rather than prevention of it, and that foundational choice shapes everything downstream. Agencies act when evidence becomes overwhelming, when headlines accumulate, when litigation threatens revenues that matter to people with influence over the process. Until those conditions are met, the burden of safety falls on families, who have no mechanism for establishing the proof the system requires and no recourse when the biology being protected absorbs the cost of the years it takes to establish it. The precautionary principle, the idea that the burden of proof should fall on those introducing a substance into the environment rather than on those exposed to it, has never been the operating logic of American chemical or food regulation. What operates instead is a tolerance-based model that asks how much harm is acceptable and answers that question in ways that consistently under-weight the interests of children and overweight the interests of industries whose products are under review.

Certain pesticides remain approved for use on food crops even after research links them to measurable IQ reductions and structural changes in children's developing brains. The research is credible, replicated, and published in peer-reviewed journals, and the regulatory response has been partial, delayed, and shaped at every stage by industry challenges to the methodology, the exposure estimates, and the threshold calculations. Chlorpyrifos stayed in use for years after the scientific case against it had solidified, and its eventual restriction came through litigation and political pressure rather than through the regulatory process working as its architects intended it to work. The children exposed during those intervening years had no appeal. Their neurodevelopment proceeded inside conditions that the system had been told were harmful and chose, for reasons that had nothing to do with their biology, to maintain.

Synthetic dyes flagged in European regulatory reviews for their association with hyperactivity and attention disruption still color American snack foods, cereals, and beverages marketed directly to children, because the American regulatory conclusion was that the evidence was inconclusive. Inconclusive is a regulatory category that does real work in this system. It means the evidence is strong enough to generate concern among scientists who've looked closely at it, but the standard of proof required to act hasn't been formally met, which allows the status quo to continue while the question is studied further, at a pace and with a funding structure that the affected industries have significant capacity to shape. Meanwhile, the children eating those dyes daily are running a longitudinal study the system was never willing to fund, and their parents are collecting the results in real time without any formal mechanism for submitting them as evidence.

Sweetened milk remains a default offering in federally funded school meal programs because it satisfies a calcium and vitamin D requirement that could be met through other means but that the dairy industry has successfully enshrined in the nutritional guidelines that shape procurement decisions. The regulatory and dietary guidance systems are downstream of the same agricultural subsidies and commodity group lobbying that determine which foods are abundant, which industries are politically powerful, and which nutritional claims receive federal endorsement. When a regulatory outcome consistently aligns with the interests of a well-funded industry and consistently diverges from the findings of independent research, the explanation worth examining is structural: a system whose inputs are shaped by the people most invested in particular outputs tends to produce those outputs, not through coordination but through the ordinary operation of incentive.

That structural dynamic is visible in personnel patterns too. Officials who shape food safety standards, pesticide tolerances, and chemical approvals move between regulatory agencies and the industries they regulate, and that movement is well-documented across administrations and decades. They bring industry perspectives into regulatory roles and regulatory expertise into industry consulting practices. The accumulated effect is a narrowing of the distance between regulator and regulated that researchers and watchdog organizations have studied and named. Whether any individual is acting in good faith matters less than what the pattern produces: a regulatory process that, across time and across administrations, tends to reach conclusions the affected industries can live with. That tendency is worth naming without overstating. It's a structural gravity, not a conspiracy, and structural gravity is in some ways harder to correct precisely because no single decision produces it.

By the time agencies act, the biology they were charged with protecting has already absorbed the cost of the delay. Neurons have been carrying a load that the system had information suggesting was harmful and chose to continue permitting. Developmental windows have narrowed inside conditions that independent science raised concerns about while the regulatory process deliberated. The children who were young during those years of deliberation are older now, and the effects of their exposures are woven into their neurodevelopment in ways that can be studied retrospectively but can't be reversed. The restriction, when it finally arrives, applies to future exposures. It can't reach back to the children whose biology was the long-running study the system was never willing to formally acknowledge.

Parents sense this timeline intuitively. They understand, often before they can articulate it, that the regulatory system operates on a clock that has no relationship to their child's developmental schedule, and they respond by making the changes they can make now rather than waiting for the official clearance that may arrive years too late to matter. A mother who reads about a pesticide concern and starts buying organic produce for her toddler before the regulatory review concludes isn't being paranoid. She's correctly reading two clocks at once: the one her child's brain is on, and the one the regulatory process is on. Those clocks have never been synchronized, and she knows which one her child is actually running on.

This is the practical reality that the protection-that-arrives-late model creates for families: the burden of early action falls on the people with the least institutional support for taking it. Families with resources can buy organic, filter water, research ingredients, and choose products based on independent safety assessments rather than regulatory approval. Families without those resources live inside the system's defaults and absorb the biological consequences of the system's delays. The regulatory failure isn't distributed evenly. It lands hardest on the children whose families have the fewest alternatives when the system's defaults turn out to be wrong.

Children's biology moves on its own schedule, indifferent to what's pending in a regulatory docket. Synapses prune. Energy systems mature. Detox pathways come online at their own developmental pace, which determines how much of a given exposure a child can clear and how much accumulates in tissue that's still building itself. The mismatch between that biological timeline and the timeline of regulatory action is where the damage lives, and it's a mismatch the system has never been structured to take seriously, because taking it seriously would require a different foundational commitment than the one American regulation is built on. It would require treating children's developing biology as the constraint that shapes permissible exposure rather than as one input among many in a cost-benefit calculation that also weights economic disruption, industry feasibility, and the political cost of acting before consensus is formally declared.

That shift hasn't happened yet. The architecture still mistakes delay for prudence and treats the absence of proof as the presence of safety. It still asks developing brains to serve as the long-running study it was never willing to fund. And it still delivers protection to children on a timeline calibrated to everything except the thing that matters most: the pace at which a young nervous system is building the architecture it'll live inside for the rest of its life.

A mother once asked how long a restriction she'd read about might take to reach her child's favorite snacks. Years, she was told. Maybe longer. She nodded, put her phone in her pocket, and stopped buying them that afternoon. That exchange lasted less than a minute and accomplished more than the regulatory process had managed in a decade. That's what it looks like when a parent correctly understands the two clocks and decides which one her child is actually on.

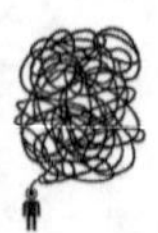

CHAPTER 35

THE QUIET REVOLUTION

EVERY PARENT MEETS a moment when the illusion cracks. Sometimes it's in a cafeteria, when you see the tray and realize it isn't a meal. Sometimes it's in a clinic, when your concern is dismissed with a handout. Sometimes it's at home, when your child spirals after a fortified snack and you finally connect the dots. The moment doesn't have to be loud. But once it arrives, it doesn't leave.

You start seeing what was always there. The system wasn't built to nourish a developing brain. It was built to move product, cut costs, stabilize markets, and quiet political pressure, and it was designed to regulate access rather than outcomes. The physiology that matters most, keeping disruption low and repair capacity high, never made the cut. That truth lands hard, and it's supposed to.

Parents have been told to wait: for better guidelines, better policies, better data. But waiting has a biological cost that accumulates with every passing day. Each day the same inputs continue, biology bends further. You don't need permission to act, and you don't need a new regulation to protect your child. You need only to see clearly what the system won't.

You aren't powerless inside this structure. As the gatekeeper of your child's inputs, your steady choices can lower disruption, raise repair capacity, and create conditions where a developing brain can recover its rhythm. You can reclaim what enters your child's body and refuse to keep outsourcing that protection to institutions that were never designed to provide it.

When enough parents act this way, the system shifts. It has to. Big Government can regulate the tray and write the legal code, but it can't regulate the persistence of a parent who sees clearly. The inputs are still yours to choose. Your child's brain is still becoming. Neuroplasticity is on your side, and the window is still open. See the cracks, and refuse to look away. That's the quiet revolution.

Do This Before Your Next Appointment

Get it in writing. Ask your child's school for its wellness or nutrition policy, and read the fine print.

Change one factor today. Pack a meal, cut one additive, move bedtime earlier.

Use this script. "My child's focus and sleep shift with food and environment. What accommodations are available?"

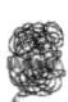

POLICY WRITES THE RULES. Big Media writes the story around them, deciding which questions sound reasonable, which concerns get filed as fringe, and which harms stay invisible because the people with platforms never thought to ask. By the time a parent arrives at a waiting room with something they've noticed and can't explain, they've already passed through a filter that shapes what they're willing to say out loud and whether they'll trust themselves enough to say it.

Big Government regulates access. Big Media regulates perception. Part Six traces how parents get trained to doubt their own eyes, and what it costs when they do.

REFERENCES

1. Abraham, J. (1995). *Science, Politics and the Pharmaceutical Industry: Controversy and Bias in Drug Regulation*. Routledge. ISBN: 978-1857282009.

2. Brownell, K. D., & Warner, K. E. (2011). The perils of ignoring history: Big Tobacco played dirty and millions died. How similar is Big Food? *Milbank Quarterly*, 87(1), 259–294. Retrieved from https://doi.org/10.1111/j.1468-0009.2009.00555.x.

3. Carpenter, D., & Moss, D. A. (2013). *Preventing Regulatory Capture: Special Interest Influence and How to Limit It*. Cambridge University Press. ISBN: 978-1107646704.

4. Eban, K. (2019). *Bottle of Lies: The Inside Story of the Generic Drug Boom*. Ecco. ISBN: 978-0062338792.

5. Michaels, D. (2020). *The Triumph of Doubt: Dark Money and the Science of Deception*. Oxford University Press.

6. Nestle, M. (2013). *Food Politics: How the Food Industry Influences Nutrition and Health* (3rd ed.). University of California Press. ISBN: 978-0520254039.

7. Nestle, M. (2018). *Unsavory Truth: How Food Companies Skew the Science of What We Eat*. Basic Books. ISBN: 978-1541697119.

8. OpenSecrets. (2024). Lobbying spending by industry: 2024. *Center for Responsive Politics*. Retrieved from https://www.opensecrets.org/federal-lobbying/industries.

9. Stiglitz, J. E. (2019). *People, Power, and Profits: Progressive Capitalism for an Age of Discontent*. W. W. Norton. ISBN: 978-1324004219.

PART 6
BIG MEDIA
A SYSTEM, NOT A SOURCE

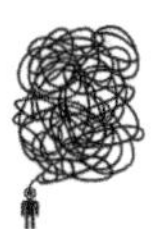

CHAPTER 36

WHEN CARE BECOMES CONTENT

A REEL OPENS to the sound of a piano. A mother speaks in nap-time light. Her daughter didn't walk until twenty months, she says. She was told not to worry, but she followed her gut. Then come the supplements that changed everything. You watch to the end without noticing, and your chest loosens. Someone refused to wait and noticed what the white coats dismissed. Someone offers what helped, just in case it helps you too. It feels like care, not manipulation. That's why it works.

What looks like empathy online is often influence disguised as intimacy: marketing wrapped in parental tone, designed to soften your center and quiet the signal that tells you something isn't right. This is Big Media. It leans in and soothes. It arrives as another parent carrying the same tired tenderness you feel at day's end, because kinship changes the math.

Old misinformation had edges. Grainy video, shouting headlines, fringe theory dressed as certainty. Now the edges blur into lowercase captions, soft rooms, and familiar cadence. Trust settles first, and the product appears later. That's the model. Platforms sell proximity. The influencer economy is built on closeness, drawing you out of the role of viewer and into something that feels like community. When she shares what worked for us, it lands like wisdom passed across a kitchen table between people who'd trade babysitting without asking. As proximity holds attention, the clock runs.

Big Media learned from marketing's early failures. The shouting stopped. Fewer claims trigger skepticism now, because more performances trigger connection instead. Instinct is mirrored, concern is validated, and care is performed while the link waits patiently in the caption. You're exhausted, dismissed after a fifteen-minute visit, alone with questions that won't quiet. Of course you search. The system counts on it.

Some parents find real things in that search. Accurate information, genuine community, a name for something they'd been watching for months without language for it. That's worth saying plainly, because dismissing every online connection would be its own distortion. The risk isn't that the internet is uniformly harmful. It's that the architecture surrounding genuine connection is optimized for something other than your child's wellbeing, and that architecture is largely invisible while you're inside it.

I once watched a father step sideways from that pull. He chose one trusted source his clinician had recommended, and when a viral protocol crossed his feed, he weighed it against that guidance rather than spiraling into the next video. He stayed steady, which is the rarest resource in most homes, and his daughter's biology followed.

Researchers who study platform design describe engagement systems that track viewing behavior and surface content calibrated to what keeps individual users watching longest. Parenting content about child struggle travels particularly well through these systems, because fear and hope are among the most reliable drivers of watch time. The result, documented across multiple platforms, is that the most emotionally activating content tends to reach the most people, regardless of its accuracy. That's a structural outcome of how engagement is measured and rewarded, and it operates the same way whether or not any individual creator intends harm. Understanding it as architecture rather than conspiracy is what makes it navigable: the problem isn't that every voice online is misleading. It's that the system surfaces the most emotionally compelling voices first, and emotional compellingness and clinical accuracy are different things that sometimes overlap and often don't.

Inside a child's body, time acts as an intervention in both directions. A week of steady sleep can calm stress pathways. A week of fragmented sleep strips resilience. Over a month, clean meals stabilize energy handling, and over that same span, heavily processed foods erode it. As the feed flickers, neurons wire to what repeats. The algorithm optimizes for return visits, not for the developing brain absorbing the cost of each detour.

Parenting content that goes viral rarely arrives as sound instruction. It arrives as memoir: emotionally textured, clinically hollow, believable enough to disarm. When the voice sounds like yours, what's absent becomes invisible. The softer the feed, the harder delay becomes to notice. You feel held, and loneliness eases. Clarity doesn't, because clarity carries friction and friction is precisely what the system removes. What remains is proximity without accountability and hope without context.

Every hour spent toggling between advice is an hour neurons wire to inconsistency. A child's brain keeps adapting while parents scroll. The algorithm steps into the space meant for a listening clinician and a steady plan, and what fills that space instead is an echo chamber engineered to keep you searching. Parents are cornered in sequence: dismissed first by the system that should have helped them, then poorly served by the one that noticed their need.

Big Media tells stories that hook. Biology writes stories that stick. The brain follows only one, and it was never following the feed.

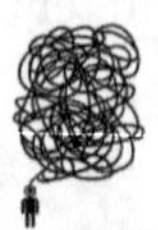

CHAPTER 37

INTIMACY BECOMES INFLUENCE

BIG MEDIA'S sophistication lies in its softness. It sits beside you, borrowing your kitchen light and your tone, telling stories that sound like your own. It asks almost nothing in return. Almost.

The parent scrolling at two in the morning has already been dismissed by the people who were supposed to listen. Their nervous system won't settle, so they search for a voice that finally acknowledges what they already sense. The algorithm is built for this moment. Intimacy becomes influence, and it begins with attention and ends with purchase, bridged entirely by proximity.

A creator calls you friend. She films at the sink, folding laundry as she talks. Your mirror neurons fire, your shoulders drop, and you feel connected. As your guard softens, the system takes note. Platform engagement systems track viewing patterns and surface more of what slows the thumb, delivering content calibrated to what keeps each user watching. Resonance stitches you to strangers who click like you do, and over time your feed narrows and nuance evaporates. What felt like discovery becomes a loop.

Creators are shaped by that loop as surely as viewers are. A post saved twice as often becomes the template for the next ten. Lighting stays warm, edges stay smooth, and claims soften toward your ache and away from the truth, because the algorithm rewards what travels emotionally rather than what holds biologically. This isn't a coordinated effort. It's what happens when engagement is the metric and emotional resonance drives engagement. Instruction used to arrive as steps. Now it arrives as a life you're invited to inhabit: a morning montage, a confession, a breakdown filmed with care and edited to music. Softness disarms and familiarity lowers resistance. You don't argue with a friend's story. You hold it. As feeling is polished, context thins. The hard parts of real intervention, repetition, monotony, and time, are traded for a reveal. Reveals travel fast. The hard parts don't.

Commerce slips in without friction. Affiliate links blend into captions, and "this is what worked for us" sits directly above a storefront. Discount codes feel like inclusion. You're no longer simply a customer. You're inside the circle, and your purchase validates her story while her story validates your hope. Hope sells. The sequence has become so practiced it's nearly invisible: proximity first, then permission, then the offer, then proof in the form of before-and-after images that are easy to feel and difficult to verify. The loop closes with a disclaimer, this isn't medical advice, language that protects the seller far more than the child. At each step, intimacy deepens as substance recedes.

A mother I worked with was awake at one in the morning after her son had screamed through bedtime. She opened her phone to escape the panic, and a creator in a soft sweater whispered about nervous system resets, then linked to a basket of oils, a weighted blanket, and a magnesium spray. The basket looked like relief, so she bought all three and fell asleep on the couch. The next morning came sharp. Her son's day started late, breakfast was sweet and rushed, and school unraveled. She cried in the garage after pickup, blaming herself for choosing wrong.

She did choose, but inside a narrowed frame. The option on

offer drew her away from the basics her child needed to land the day: sunlight, protein first, water, an earlier night in a darker room. These are small, unglamorous moves that look insignificant until you stack them across weeks, and they're precisely the moves the system passes over because they can't be monetized. That's the tell. What holds attention spreads faster than what restores a child's capacity, and stickiness beats steadiness because the platform was never designed to care about the difference.

Many stories feel true enough to trust, and some of the mechanisms they describe are real. But healing makes a demand most stories can't meet. A child's brain changes when stabilizing conditions are held long enough to matter, repeated, predictable, and sustained over time rather than revealed in an instant. The harm in trying what you see online isn't always obvious, especially when the science sounds right. It lies in assuming that a child on a screen matches your child's biology. Similar stories suggest shared nervous systems and shared thresholds. They don't. What helps one child can overstimulate another. What steadies one nervous system can strain a different one. What supports repair in one body can quietly add burden in another, because healing happens in context, and removing that context means even well-intended ideas can cause harm.

Online content can explain mechanisms, orient attention, and name possibilities worth exploring. What it can't do is individualize risk, account for the total load a child is already carrying, or see the thresholds and trade-offs that determine whether an intervention helps or quietly adds to the strain. Without those, even well-meant guidance can tip a fragile system in the wrong direction. A child's brain adapts to context, not intent, and the feed has never been able to see the context it can't film.

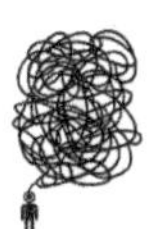

CHAPTER 38

DELAY ISN'T NEUTRAL

THERE'S a kind of knowing that lives below language, the part of you that registered the change in your child before you had words for it, that felt the shift in a laugh or a gaze or a sleep pattern before any of it was nameable. That knowing was your most accurate instrument. Then the feed got hold of it. One expert contradicted another. One thread reframed what you'd observed as something else entirely. One caption arrived at exactly the right moment of exhaustion and offered a story that was easier to hold than the one your body was telling you. And the inner pulse, the one calibrated to your specific child across years of daily proximity, began to feel less certain than the voices accumulating in your phone.

That erosion is the product. Delay arrives dressed as information, as community, as the reasonable suggestion that you gather more data before you act. Each piece of content that reframes your urgency as overreaction, that recasts regression as individuality, that softens a pattern of loss into a portrait of a child breaking a mold, registers in the nervous system as a low-grade threat that never fully resolves. Planning circuits quiet as protective circuits take over. The scroll continues not because you're weak but because the system was built to hold attention, and a frightened parent's attention is among the most persistent it can find.

The algorithm doesn't know your child. It knows your behavior: which posts made you slow your thumb, which captions made your breath catch, which stories you watched to the end at two in the morning when you should've been sleeping. Recommendation systems surface content based on engagement patterns, and engagement patterns for parents of struggling children tend to cluster around fear, hope, and the space between them. Retention is the metric. Your child's developmental trajectory is invisible to it, and the gap between what the system is optimizing for and what you actually need is precisely where the damage from delay accumulates.

When action stalls, the nervous system shifts into scanning mode. Sustained uncertainty is a physiological state before it's an emotional one, and cortisol that should spike and resolve instead idles, maintaining a low-grade vigilance that gradually degrades the cognitive capacities you need most: the ability to recognize a pattern clearly, hold a plan in mind, and take the next step without being derailed by the next contradictory voice. Attention lingers longest in the space between alarm and relief, and a business model built on lingering attention has no structural incentive to resolve that space. So it doesn't.

A mother arrived at a clinical visit carrying a binder thick with printed protocols, supplement schedules, and forum threads. She'd been researching for eight months. Her son was two years and four months old, and in those eight months his language had plateaued, his sleep had fragmented further, and the eye contact that had been inconsistent was now rare. She was visibly depleted, shallow breath and flat tone, the particular exhaustion of someone who's been working very hard in a direction that hasn't been helping. She said she didn't know what to do next. What she meant was that she'd lost confidence in her own knowing, because eight months of conflicting information had taught her to distrust it. The binder was evidence of effort and evidence of paralysis simultaneously. She'd been consuming instead of acting, and the system that sold her the consumption had no interest in telling her the difference.

Her son's biology had kept moving.

At two years and four months, the language window that peaks in the second year was already narrowing. Synaptic pruning proceeds according to a biological schedule that has no relationship to how long it takes to find consensus online, and no consensus exists online anyway, only competing claims calibrated to different fears. Every week she'd spent in the binder was a week her son's nervous system had continued wiring itself around the conditions it was living inside: fragmented sleep, fuel instability from a diet she'd been adjusting on conflicting advice, and the ambient stress of a household organized around a child's struggle rather than around the steadiness that struggling child most needed. The delay had a biological address, and it was in her son's developing brain.

In the first thousand days of a child's life, the brain forms connections at a rate that will never be matched again, over a million new synaptic connections per second at peak periods of growth, each one requiring the right inputs to form correctly, to stabilize, and to survive the pruning process that determines which circuits persist into later development. The inputs those connections depend on are mundane: stable fuel, deep sleep, low inflammatory burden, predictable sensory experience, and the responsive social engagement that language and connection circuits are built from. When those inputs are disrupted, connections form around the disruption rather than despite it, and those adaptations have structural consequences that extend far beyond the period when they were made.

Sleep fragmented through the second year doesn't produce a child who's simply tired. Sleep is when the brain consolidates what it learned during waking hours, when metabolic waste is cleared from neural tissue, when stress chemistry resets, and when the slow-wave activity that supports memory formation and synaptic refinement occurs. A child who spends months in that fragmented state is a child whose brain is being asked to build without adequate time for construction, and the result is a nervous system that's adapted to operating without the restoration it was designed to require, changing its baseline in ways that addressing sleep debt alone can't fully reverse. Fuel instability compounds the same problem through a different mechanism. The developing brain is disproportionately sensitive to the volatility that refined carbohydrates and sweetened drinks produce. Spikes and crashes disrupt the electrochemical environment that synaptic transmission depends on, alter neurotransmitter availability, and trigger stress chemistry that keeps the nervous system in a state of low-grade vigilance that competes directly with the learning and social engagement development requires. A month of that isn't background noise. It's biology bending.

A mother noticed her son's babbling had faded at thirteen months. The sounds that had been building toward words had quieted, and the turn-taking that typically precedes language was harder to elicit. Her pediatrician suggested he was likely focused on motor development, a common pattern, and recommended monitoring. She went home and opened her phone. A reel told her he wasn't behind, he was breaking the mold. A thread told her boys are just slower. A podcast told her that the push to hit language milestones was itself a form of anxiety that she should examine. Each of these voices was wrong, but each was compelling in the specific way that content calibrated to parental fear is compelling: it offered relief from urgency at the exact moment urgency was the appropriate response.

She waited. The babbling didn't return. At eighteen months there was less sound than there'd been at thirteen. At twenty months there were long stretches of quiet that she now understood weren't contemplative but absent, a nervous system that had reduced output because maintaining it had become too costly. Therapy began after diagnosis, but the language window had narrowed in the intervening months, and the circuits that build most readily in the second year build more slowly and with more effort after it. Plasticity remained, as it always does, but the margin for repair had thinned. What the feed had cost her wasn't a missed appointment. It was seven months of a developmental window she'd been persuaded to wait through.

Each new piece of content hints at resolution and opens another question. Certainty would stop the scroll, so the architecture produces everything except certainty, because certainty ends the engagement and engagement is what the model monetizes. Confidence goes the same way as urgency. The parent who once trusted her own noticing begins to doubt it, losing access to the precision because the feed has introduced enough competing interpretations of every signal that the signal itself becomes unreadable. Coherence goes first, then agency, and the system benefits from both losses because a parent who's lost confidence in their own knowing is a parent who needs more content.

The exit isn't dramatic. It's a decision made once and then maintained against the pull of a system that'll keep trying to draw you back. One trusted source, recommended by a clinician who knows your child, replaces the feed as the reference point for questions that arise. Observations get recorded and brought to appointments rather than typed into search bars at midnight. The inner pulse, the one that registered the change before language arrived for it, gets treated as data rather than as a symptom of anxiety to be soothed by consumption. Action gets taken on the biological timeline rather than on the timeline the content cycle runs on, because those two timelines serve different interests and your child's development is served by only one of them.

The system profits from not yet. Your child's brain has never had the luxury of waiting, and the distance between those two facts is the most important thing the feed will never tell you.

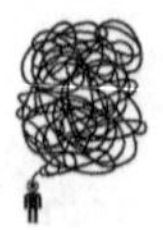

CHAPTER 39

YOUR NOTICING IS DATA

THE PART of you that's been searching is awake. Your nervous system is doing what it was built to do: track, protect, and adapt. The problem isn't that you don't know enough. It's that you've been taught to distrust what you already know.

You're overloaded and exhausted from metabolizing too many contradictions. But beneath the noise, you still notice the way your child's skin feels when something is off. You know the difference between a tantrum and a cry that comes from deep inside the body. You notice when their eyes lose focus, when their breath changes, or when the spark dims for reasons no one else can name. That awareness isn't anxiety. It's biology.

Mirror neurons fire when you track their movement. Oxytocin rises when you hold them. Your circuits shift to match theirs, calibrating to every cue in real time. You're collecting data the way the body always has, through presence, through proximity, through the kind of sustained attention that no algorithm can replicate. That's embodied expertise, a living feedback loop between two nervous systems designed to read each other across years of daily contact.

Big Media wants you to outsource that knowing. It floods the channel until your inner signal sounds like static, training you to believe that certainty belongs to someone else: the influencer who says detox, the thread that says calm down, the caption that reframes your urgency as overreaction. It prizes consumption over truth and engagement over steadiness, and it profits most when you trust it more than you trust yourself. That's the transaction, and it was never in your child's interest.

Stay with what you notice. Most early shifts, the sleep regression, the blank stare, the laugh that turns brittle, surface before tests show anything and before doctors agree on labels. You sense them because your biology and your child's are entangled in a way that no platform can access and no feed can approximate. When a system dismisses that data, the system is the one in need of repair.

One parent told me she stopped following parenting accounts, stopped comparing routines, and started protecting three things: daylight, breakfast, and bedtime. Within months, her son's tantrums shortened. Within a year, her own headaches eased. Nothing dramatic, just biology stabilizing once the interference lifted. That's what the feed can't sell, because it doesn't scale. Stability doesn't require new content every day. It doesn't keep you scrolling. It grounds you in pattern, in body, and in what's actually real, and that groundedness is precisely what Big Media's business model depends on you never finding.

Step out of the swirl, and the contradiction quiets. You stop chasing fixes outside and start hearing the ones inside. You act from experience, choosing one next right thing and doing it long enough for cells to notice. No algorithm knows your child the way you do. No platform can see what you've seen across years of daily proximity, and no feed can replicate the diagnostic precision of a parent who has been paying attention since the beginning.

The system will try to convince you that consumption is caring. It wins when you ignore your own data. You already hold the information that matters most. Trust it, and the system loses its hold. The noise will persist: headlines, hashtags, and confident strangers with links in their bios. Let them pass. And the next time someone tells you to wait, remind them that biology doesn't.

Do This Before Your Next Appointment

One trusted source. Choose a single reputable place for health guidance. Write it down. Example options: American Academy of Pediatrics, National Institutes of Health, Mayo Clinic.

One myth check. Note the most alarming claim you've seen this week. Before you share it, run it past your chosen source.

Use this script. "I've read X online. Can you help me understand whether this applies to my child?"

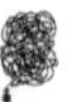

YOU'VE SEEN the whole architecture now. Each system doing its part, none of them requiring a villain, all of them producing the same outcome: a child's biology bending under pressure that gets called normal, a parent's knowing getting filed as anxiety, and a machinery that mistakes collapse for coincidence because coincidence is easier to sustain than accountability.

The way through has always been simpler than the systems

want it to be. Steadiness, supply, safety, and time. Biology has recognized these things long before any of the five systems existed, and it recognizes them still. Clarity comes first. Then repair. They've always moved in that order, and now that you can see what you're up against, they can finally move together.

REFERENCES

1. Alter, A. (2017). *Irresistible: The Rise of Addictive Technology and the Business of Keeping Us Hooked*. Penguin Press. ISBN: 978-1594206641.
2. Eyal, N. (2014). *Hooked: How to Build Habit-Forming Products*. Portfolio/Penguin. ISBN: 978-1591847786.
3. Haidt, J. (2023). *The Anxious Generation: How the Great Rewiring of Childhood Is Causing an Epidemic of Mental Illness*. Penguin Press. ISBN: 978-0593655030.
4. Khoo, K., et al. (2008). Health information seeking by parents in the Internet age. *Journal of Pediatrics and Child Health, 44*, 419–423. Retrieved from https://doi.org/10.1111/j.1440-1754.2008.01322.x.
5. Kramer, A. D. I., et al. (2014). Experimental evidence of massive-scale emotional contagion through social networks. *Proceedings of the National Academy of Sciences, 111*(24), 8788–8790. Retrieved from https://doi.org/10.1073/pnas.1320040111.
6. Lazer, D. M. J., et al. (2018). The science of fake news. *Science, 359*(6380), 1094–1096. Retrieved from https://doi.org/10.1126/science.aao2998.
7. Lustig, R. H. (2017). *The Hacking of the American Mind: The Science Behind the Corporate Takeover of Our Bodies and Brains*. Avery. ISBN: 978-1101982587.
8. Pariser, E. (2011). *The Filter Bubble: What the Internet Is Hiding from You*. Penguin Press. ISBN: 978-1594203008.
9. Vosoughi, S., et al. (2018). The spread of true and false news online. *Science, 359*(6380), 1146–1151. Retrieved from https://doi.org/10.1126/science.aap9559.

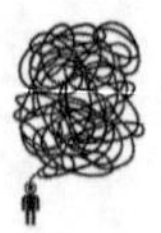

EPILOGUE

THE DAY THE NOISE STOPPED

IT BEGAN WITHOUT CEREMONY. No vow, no plan, no announcement. Just morning.

The phone lay facedown on the counter. Light through the kitchen window looked ordinary, maybe softer. A child's bowl waited while water ran. The house felt less like something to manage and more like something alive. No new protocol waited in the inbox, no headline to decode, no voice naming the next fear. The silence felt foreign. Then holy.

For months, she'd measured safety by noise: the next story, the next parent who sounded sure. Quiet had meant danger and action had meant scrolling. She hadn't realized how completely the algorithm had colonized her instincts. Without it, her body began to recalibrate. Her breath deepened before her mind caught up. Her pulse, once synced to the rhythm of notifications, found a slower meter. This was the body remembering how to listen to itself.

Her son padded in, hair still wild from sleep, and climbed into the chair beside her. No fuss, no rush, just the rhythm of spoon against bowl. Every cell registered the shift as the noise thinned.

Questions remained, as they always would. But they no

longer pressed like alarms. Questions had become coordinates pointing her toward what mattered next rather than weapons turning her against herself. She'd spent years waiting for systems to do what they were designed to avoid: change. They hadn't. But in the quiet, she saw what the noise had hidden: one nervous system refusing to abandon another.

That's where repair began.

The child looked up, mouth full of oatmeal, and smiled. It was a small, unguarded moment, with nothing viral about it, and yet it held everything the systems had missed: stability, connection, oxygen, and safety. Presence marked the threshold, because the brain repairs what it can perceive and builds around what it can't. Once observation replaced panic, she could see again: her child, her own hands, and the difference between motion and care.

Outside, the air smelled clean, and she noticed. That was the beginning. The day the noise stopped was the day reality became visible.

The systems hadn't fallen. They were still out there, humming with distortion and distraction, but their hold had broken. She no longer mistook volume for truth. She kept the apps and kept the doctors and kept the science. She simply stopped handing them her nervous system and her child's future.

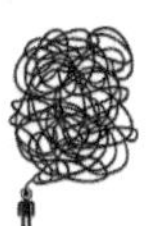

AFTERWORD

THE CAVALRY ISN'T COMING

They promised the cavalry was coming. A breakthrough drug, new guidelines, a better therapy, and policy reform that would finally safeguard children. You waited, complied, and trusted. Still, your child's body unraveled.

This book exposed what breaks the brain: five systems that promise protection and deliver erosion. Big Food destabilizes. Big Pharma sedates. Big Medicine fragments. Big Government delays. Big Media distorts. Each part of this book peeled back a layer of trust you were taught to outsource, and together they forced one conclusion: a child can't develop inside a hierarchy that sidelines truth.

You've seen injury stack until defenses fray. You've seen data pile up without ownership, delaying action as capacity slips. You've seen waiting consume time the brain can't spare. The systems you were told to lean on were built to manage, not to restore, and the questions that follow from that recognition press in hard.

If the cavalry wasn't built to arrive in time, the answers have to live somewhere else. They always have. In movement, sleep, nutrients, and calm. In the basics dismissed as secondary because they can't be patented, packaged, or scaled. In the fundamentals that belong to you, and through you, to your child. Biology has always responded to these inputs. The systems simply learned to make you forget that.

The antidote to broken systems has always been clarity. Clarity about what the body needs, what the systems provide, and the distance between those two things. You've traveled that distance across every chapter of this book. You know what you're looking at now.

So: if not them, then who?

You.

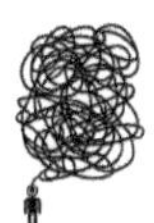

ACKNOWLEDGMENTS

To Aiden and Lexi, my children, who are my reason and my teachers. Every inch of clarity I carry was earned through loving you and learning from you.

To the parents who trusted me with their stories. You questioned what was presented as settled. You kept going when systems asked you to wait, to soften, or to doubt yourselves. This book carries your courage and your persistence.

To the clinicians and allied professionals who practice with curiosity and humility, even inside systems that reward speed over understanding. You remind me, daily, that integrity still lives in medicine.

Thank you.

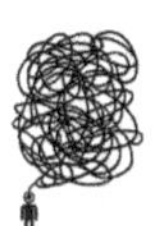

ABOUT THE AUTHOR

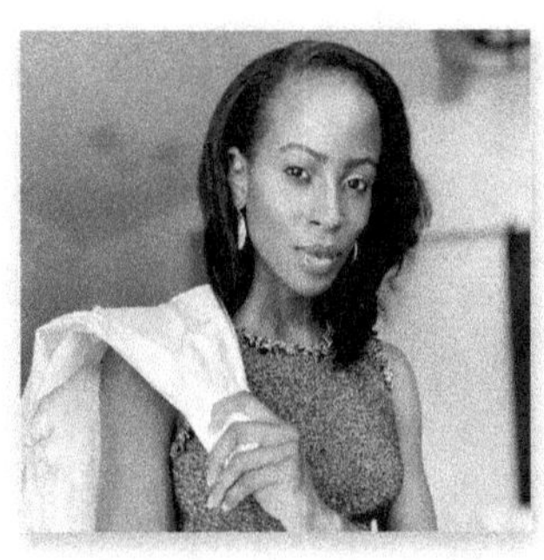

Dr. Kimberly Idoko is a Yale-, Penn-, Columbia-, and Stanford-educated neurologist and attorney who works with families navigating neurodevelopmental differences. She brings a rare combination of clinical neuroscience, systems literacy, and lived experience as a mother to the question parents are rarely given time to ask: what is actually happening inside my child's brain?

She is a board-certified physician who cares for thousands of patients each year. She is also the founder of Special Parent Coach, where she helps parents interpret early neurological signs and understand how modern systems shape outcomes. She lives in Los Angeles with her family.

drkimberlyidoko.substack.com
instagram.com/drkimberlyidoko
tiktok.com/@drkimberlyidoko